WHY ANIMAL$

~ And How Low-Carb and Paleo Diets Sicken and Kill Us ~

Book 3 - Summary:
Deficiencies and Consequences

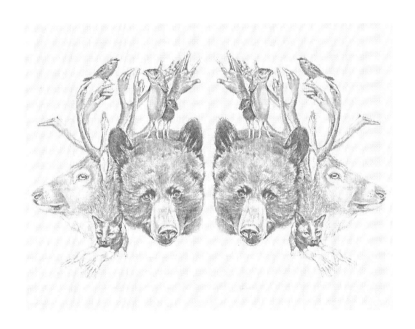

Rohan Millson

Tabularasa Press
Cape Town 2016

DISCLAIMER

The information contained in this book is for educational purposes only and is not intended to be, and should not be used by you as medical advice. **Please DO NOT delay in seeking medical advice from a licensed health care professional for any health problems you may experience. Please DO NOT base any health care decision on the information contained in this book**, no matter how strongly the author believes the evidence shows that lifestyle medicine and preventive whole-food, plants-only nutrition are the best remedy for most chronic ailments.

What people are saying about *Why Animals Aren't Food*

"With passion, wit, and facts, Rohan Millson shows why choosing to eat animals isn't bad only for them, and exposes the irony that when we rob them of their lives, we raise the risk of doing the same to ourselves."

- **Jonathan Balcombe**, PhD, author of *Pleasurable Kingdom* and *What a Fish Knows*

"Rohan is passionate about health that is honest and true and this book is an honest approach to the truth about human nutrition - we all need to read this - it can change our lives and make the world a better place."

- **Mary-Ann Shearer**, founder of The Natural Way

"This remarkable book not only summarizes the nutritional discoveries that can liberate us from the abuse that animal foods inflict on our physical health, it explains and catalogues them with an astonishing degree of depth and breadth. Anyone of us who takes the time to read and understand the empowering information contained in this book will learn how we can live more healthy and productive lives, and contribute to a more harmonious world."

- **Will Tuttle**, PhD, author of *The World Peace Diet*

"One day every enslaved animal will obtain their freedom and the animal rights movement will succeed because no lie can live forever. As an in-the-trenches activist for nearly 20 years, I tried EVERYTHING in my power - from direct action and civil disobedience to education and advertising - to make people understand that animals have been victimized to such a degree that they aren't even considered to be victims. They aren't even considered at all. Humans have actually turned animals into inanimate objects; sandwiches and shoes. But animals are not food, clothing, entertainment or research specimens under any circumstance!

Rohan Millson, with his extraordinary book *Why Animals Aren't Food*, is doing everything in his power, as well, to expose the lies and help us understand why animals should play no part in the human diet."

- **Gary Yourofsky**, founder of ADAPTT, Animals Deserve Absolute Protection Today and Tomorrow

COPYRIGHT ACKNOWLEDGMENTS

ISBN-13: 978-1530222612
ISBN-10: 1530222613

Cover art: Details from "Kohler's Pig," with kind permission of the artist,
copyright Michael Sowa 2016

Cover design: Mark van Wyk (http://earthalive.org)

Frontispiece: "Hybrid I," with kind permission of the artist,
copyright Oriana Fenwick 2016

Many thanks to all the cartoonists and other artists who've given their
permission to reprint their work in this book.

Special thanks for their generous support to

Dan Piraro of Bizarro.com for his brilliant cartoons
Michael Sowa for the evocative front cover image
Oriana Fenwick for the quirky frontispiece
Mary-Ann and Mark Shearer
Mark and Tarryn van Wyk
Will and Madeleine Tuttle
The Ghost of Brooklyn
Andre Phillipe Côté
Dr. Michael Greger
Evolve! Campaigns
Dr. Neal Barnard
VeganStreet.com
Nicola Vernon
Michael Haupt
John Darkow
Steve Sack
PCRM

No animals were harmed during the 5 years it took to make this book. 49 were adopted.

DEDICATION

I dedicate this book to Michael Greger, Will Tuttle and Nicola Vernon, crazy diamonds of the first water, who personify the beautiful difference between love of animals and love of food.

Contents

Segue from Book 2 of *Why Animals Aren't Food* (~~Food~~borne Pathogens & Pollutants)   iv

Part 4 (Missing in Action)   578

Animal MIAs – Animal Deficiencies   579

Part 5 (Summary): Why Animals Aren't Food   628

When the Cows Come Home to Roost: Consequences of Meating   629

References: Landmarks in medical and nutrition research   631

A Turd's Eye View of an Animal Meal   696

On Silver Bullets & Coffin Nails   728

The Pointlessness of Meating   730

Meating and Earth's Climate   736

The Good News   741

Acknowledgments   743

"What's next?" and "Staying in touch"   745

Table of Contents - Book 3   749

Index to *Why Animals Aren't Food* (complete book)   757

About my next book, *The Low-Carb Bullshit Artists Are Lying Us to Death*   777

Segue from Book 2 of *Why Animals Aren't Food*
(~~Food~~borne Pathogens & Pollutants)

Ah, there you are. This link from Book 2 to Book 3 is to bring us all up to speed with what's in Books 1 and 2 of *Why Animals Aren't Food*, for those who haven't read them or for those who'd like a swift recap. It doesn't appear in the complete edition of the book.

In Book 1 of *Why Animals Aren't Food* we saw that

• Intrinsically, animals aren't food. They cause us too much damage when we eat them. They're made out of dozens of substances that are harmful to us. Even the proteins in animals aren't safe for humans to eat. Animal proteins acidify us with their excess sulfur-containing amino acids; they stimulate our livers to produce IGF-1, a growth hormone associated with rapid cell growth, aging and cancer; they damage our kidneys with their heavy nitrogen load; and they initiate auto-immune responses in us because they're too similar to human proteins for our immune systems to tell them apart, a dysfunctional mechanism known as molecular mimicry or, less formally, as 'friendly fire.'

Book 1 describes dozens of other animal components that sicken us and shorten our lives, including:

AGEs (a.k.a. advanced glycation end-products, glycotoxins or gerontotoxins); alpha-gal; ammonia; amyloid; arachidonic acid; benzopyrene; biogenic amines; cadaverine; casein; casomorphin; ceramide; animal copper; cysteine; diacyl-glycerol; endocrine disruptors (EDs); endotoxins; estradiol; other estrogens; galactose; harmane; heme iron; heterocyclic amines; hydrogen sulfide; IQ4,5b; lactose; lauric acid; leucine; MeIQx; methionine; myoglobin; Neu5Gc; nitrites; nitrosamines and nitrosamides; PhIP; animal phosphorus; polycyclic aromatic hydrocarbons (PAHs); purge; animal purines; putrescine; spermidine; spermine; steroid hormones; sulfur-containing amino acids; taurine; uric acid and xeno-autoantibodies.

I won't repeat them here, but there are dozens of mechanisms by which Meating sickens and kills us. I list and explain them in Book 1, which also contains a section showing how Meating causes most of the chronic degenerative conditions that send us to hospital beds or to our graves. Called by some "diseases", we now know that they're symptoms of the underlying lifestyles or behavior patterns I call Meating and Junking. Not diseases, they're elective conditions, brought on and promoted mainly by what we elect to eat.

Examples from Book 1, chosen from almost 200 Meater and, to a lesser extent, Junker "diseases", include:

acne, Alzheimer's, breast cancer, cataracts, diverticulitis, erectile dysfunction, (non-alcoholic) fatty liver disease, gallstones, hypertension, insulin resistance, jaundice, kidney stones, lupus, multiple sclerosis, non-Hodgkin's lymphoma, osteoporosis, Parkinson's, prostate cancer, quinsy, rheumatoid arthritis, SIDS (or crib death), stroke, types 1 and 2 diabetes, ulcerative colitis, urinary tract infections, varicose veins, wrinkled skin, syndrome x (a.k.a. metabolic syndrome), yeast infections and zoönoses (animal-borne infectious diseases). In fact, Book 1 showed that they're all animal-borne infectious diseases.

In Book 2 of *Why Animals Aren't Food* we saw that

- Easily 90% of the germs 'n' worms that kill us by the tens of thousands invade our bodies via the animals we eat. Part 2 (Pathogens) contains a detailed discussion of disease-causing fecal bacteria, viruses, parasitic flukes and worms, prions and other animal-borne nasties.

The Meater bacteria that can sicken and kill us include:

Bacillus cereus; *Brucella*; *Campylobacter*; *Clostridium botulinum*; *Clostridium difficile*; *Clostridium perfringens*; *Enterococcus*; *Escherichia coli* (*E. coli*); *Listeria monocytogenes*; *Mycobacterium bovis* (bovine TB); *Proteus mirabilis*; *Salmonella*; *Shigella*; *Staphylococcus aureus* and MRSA (Methicillin- or multi-drug-resistant *Staphylococcus aureus*); *Streptococcus*; *Vibrio cholerae*; *Vibrio vulnificus* (the flesh-eating bacterium); *Vibrio parahaemolyticus*; and *Yersinia enterocolitica*.

The Meater viruses that can sicken us, help fatten us and kill us include:

adenovirus 36 (an obesogenic virus); astrovirus; avian leukosis/ sarcoma virus; bovine leukemia virus; fish viruses; hepatitis A virus; hepatitis E; human papilloma virus (HPV); Marek's disease virus; norovirus; oncogenic, or cancer-causing viruses; porcine endogenous retroviruses; poultry viruses; rabies; reticuloendotheliosis virus; rotavirus; sapovirus; and wart viruses.

Plants contain these often-deadly disease vectors only when they've been cross-contaminated with animal feces.

- Part 3 (Pollutants) shows that at least 90% of the chemical contaminants that corrupt our bodies and help destroy us come from the animals we eat. The individual chemical poisons (or classes of chemicals that contain many poisons), which I listed in the "Segue to Book 3" at the end of Book 2, add up to more than 100 names. To list all the roughly 100,000 chemicals we humans spew out into the environment each year by the gigaton would fill an entire book at least twice the length of this one.

Sadly for the organic life forms on planet Earth, most persistent organic pollutants, or POPs, are lipophilic, meaning they're 'fat-loving.' They bio-accumulate in the fat of small animals, particularly fishes, which may then be eaten by larger fishes, until humans behave like peak predators and eat the largest fishes of all, like salmons and tunas, which have biomagnified deadly POPs in their fat to extraordinary levels.

That's why Meating is the most relevant source of neurotoxic, obesogenic, diabetogenic, oncogenic, teratogenic, endocrine disrupting environmental pollutants in our bodies.

And that gives us a nodding acquaintance with Books 1 and 2 of *Why Animals Aren't Food*.

In this third book, Part 4 (Missing in Action) confirms animals' unsuitability as food for humans by showing how they're deficient in just about any substance that's beneficial to us, while containing excessive amounts of stuff that's bad for us. In anatomy, form follows function - the shape of things is determined by what they do. With animals-as-food, dysfunction follows lack of form; meaning that because animals lack dozens of beneficial substances, they're also lacking in beneficial metabolic mechanisms which rely on those substances for their being.

For example, animals and junk are both hopelessly deficient in fiber (and associated nutrients, like phytates), and that makes it impossible for Meaters and Junkers to have optimal gut flora or optimal gut immune function. Only whole plants supply fiber and the other phytonutrients necessary for good bowel function. That's part of the reason why Meaters and Junkers are so much more prone to constipation and IBDs - inflammatory bowel "diseases" such as Crohn's and ulcerative colitis - and why M&Js are also far more prone to colorectal cancer. We are what we don't excrete.

The next section may be my favorite. Called "References: Landmarks in medical and nutrition research," it supplies 70-odd pages of evidence reaffirming why animals and junk aren't food, and why whole plants are. In it I cite and comment on scores of the greatest nutrition and biomedical papers ever written. Not for nothing are they called landmarks.

Strange then that the Low-Carb Bullshit Artists appear to be too myopic to have read them; which is about as believable as pretending we can't see Jørn Utzon's iconic Opera House when we're standing on top of the Sydney Harbour Bridge.

After that, I switch gears from reductionism to wholism. In "A Turd's Eye View of an Animal Meal," I do my best to explain Meating's ill-effects on our digestive tracts and our metabolisms, by following a piece of animal from the moment we put it into our mouths to the moment we excrete what remains, describing the multiple injuries it causes along the way.

That done, a Meater reader would have to be in serious denial still to believe that animals are food for human beings.

Book 3 continues with a discussion of the Consequences of Meating, for our individual physical, psychological and spiritual health, as well as for the health of human (and other sentient animal) societies and the environment. I end with The Good News, showing how beautiful existence is for Planters, and suggesting how beautiful existence could be for all of us, if we were to rediscover what is and what isn't food.

I can't tell you how good The Good News of Planting is: it's sublime, almost numinous.

I hope, if you're not already there, that you'll join us. We are the least exclusive, most welcoming club in the world. Anyone can join, any time.

As June Jordan wrote in her 'Poem for South African Women,' which she recited before the United Nations general assembly on the 9th of August, 1978:

"We are the ones we've been waiting for."

PS Following the index at the end of this book, beginning on page 777, there's a bonus chapter to introduce you to my next book, *The Low-Carb Bullshit Artists Are Lying Us to Death.*

Part 4 (Missing in Action)

Animal MIAs – Animal Deficiencies

Daniel 5:27: "Thou art weighed in the balances, and art found wanting."

In Part 1 (Animals, Themselves), we saw that *all* the natural 'ingredients' of animals are naturally inimical to our health when we eat them.

In Part 2 (~~Food~~borne Pathogens), we saw that, besides inflicting zoönotic diseases on us, animals play host to dozens of species of micro-organisms and parasites that harm our health (except the bacteria that make B_{12}!)

In Part 3 (~~Food~~borne Contaminants), we saw that – through no fault of their own – animals bio-accumulate and bio-magnify thousands of environmental toxins to thousands of times the ambient concentrations, and harm our health when we eat them.

Not only do animals cause an endless litany of ill-effects, they crucially lack the following vital components and effects provided only by plants. These are the animal Missing in Action, which re-re-confirm that we are Planters:

50 Animal Deficiencies That Rule Them Out as Food

1. Water

Without knowing it, Meaters are often chronically dehydrated. First, the fluids – blood and lymph et al – are systematically drained from animals' bodies at slaughter. *All* slaughtered animals die the same way, by bleeding to death, while they're still conscious. Blood makes animal flesh soggy and unpalatable, and it's anathema to humans, except for outliers such as the Maa-speaking Maasai and Samburu pastoralists of East Africa.

Also, Meaters tend to cook animal flesh over high, dry heat until most of the moisture is gone – there's not much water, even in the juiciest of steaks. For this and other reasons such as avoiding the carcinogens and gerontotoxins produced by cooking flesh, animals are most healthily prepared over low, moist heat in stews and soups.

To be a Meater is to be dehydrated (and constipated).

2. Chlorophyll

Chlorophyll is incredible stuff. My mind boggles when I consider chlorophyll.

In the process known as photosynthesis, or 'making from light,' plants, algae and cyanobacteria use pigments to convert the sun's energy into chemical energy. They're called photoautotrophs, which means 'light-self-feeders.' Chlorophylls of various kinds are the pigments involved.

The plants take in carbon dioxide and water from the air and soil (nitrogen too), and, using solar energy to power the reaction, they create sugar and oxygen. Energy is stored in the sugar structures and later converted into molecules of ATP (adenosine triphosphate), our cells' energy currency.

The initial chemical reaction looks like this:

$$6CO_2 + 6H_2O \rightarrow C_6H_{12}O_6 + 6O_2$$

Carbon dioxide + water $\rightarrow$ sugar + oxygen

Plants are like solar arrays, with their chlorophyll-green leaves like phyto-solar panels pointed at the sun. They absorb the sun's rays and create sugar from carbon dioxide and water, and they exhale oxygen.

And then we come along, and we eat the sugar and breathe the oxygen – the two substances that fuel humans – and we breathe out carbon dioxide and pee out water – the two substances that fuel plants. And around and around the cycle goes, humans and plants in perfect synergy.

We humans are essentially solar-powered beings. Plants are the primary solar beings, the phyto-photo-auto-trophs. We're the secondary solar beings, powered by plants.

It's so beautiful, it makes me tear up sometimes when I think about it: us and nature in perfect, peaceful harmony… going around and around, them feeding us, us feeding them in an indefinitely sustainable partnership. (Understanding our nature as solar beings makes one understand a little clearer why Meating is such an abomination – a rending asunder of our perfect human-plant relationship.)

I mentioned nitrogen above. Plants absorb nitrogen from root bacteria which 'fix' the nitrogen for them, and plants then create the amino acids that make up the proteins that make up their leaves and stems and tubers. Plants also make fats and carbohydrates. Hydrated carbon = carbon + water, essentially – a convenient storage form of glucose, our universal power molecule.

Earlier I showed a diagram comparing the structures of chlorophyll and heme, the metalloprotein in hemoglobin which carts oxygen around in our blood. Isn't this miraculous? Plants use this molecule to create oxygen out of sunlight and carbon dioxide, and then we humans adapt the same molecule to ferry our oxygen fuel (and our carbon dioxide wastes) around inside ourselves. If we get this – really get it; understand to our core that we humans developed after billions of years in inseparable association with plants – then we know with absolute certainty that we're obviously and exclusively adapted to eating nothing but plants… who, in turn, developed inseparably from cyanobacteria and algae, yet other solar-powered beings.

In this direction lies our angel nature, in Pure Planting. Eating animals is our "fundamental debacle," upsetting the perfection of the energy cycle between humans and plants and bacteria and the sun: it's inefficient, cruel, selfish and spectacularly unnecessary. Meating is beyond pointless. For solar-powered beings to power ourselves by eating the bodies of other solar-powered beings is demonic.

Besides creating the human macronutrients – carbs, fats and proteins – plants also give us the micronutrients. Plants make all the vitamins, except for B_{12} – I told you we were partners with the bacteria! – and vitamin D – I told you we were solar powered beings! Plants serve up our minerals for us too, absorbing them from the soil and making them bioavailable to us in Goldilocks amounts. Organic minerals are different to inorganic rocks (which is what table salt is – pulverized rocks which we over-consume in deadly quantities).

As we'll see in the next entry (Phytonutrients) plant pigments, usually found in plant skins and peels, are the healthiest, most antioxidant parts of plants. They're the plants' chemical sunblock and raincoat, all in one.

Besides making our food, giving us life, the phytonutrient known as chlorophyll has one other spectacular property: it's a **carcinogen interceptor**. Chlorophyll binds to carcinogens, changing their shape and preventing them from slipping into our DNA and mutating it. That's just one of the many reasons why people who eat the most plants have the lowest cancer rates. Chlorophyll prevents what Meating causes. Isn't that amazing?

There's zero chlorophyll in animals. There's nothing amazing about Meating. Meating is a chlorophyll deficiency disease.

In the first two Meater deficiencies we've covered so far, we've met the three real macronutrients: water, air and sunlight. That's what we're made out of: water, air and sunlight. Without these three, life as we know it is impossible. Meating is deficient in water, in air and in sun power.

3. Synergistic phytonutrients

OK, saying that animals lack phytonutrients isn't saying much. As we know, the 'phyto' in phytonutrients or phytochemicals or phytoestrogens merely means 'plant,' so it shouldn't gobsmack us that there aren't many in animals – less than 1/64th on average. Here's the big hairy but, though, and it's enormous: there are estimated to be more than 100,000 phytochemicals all acting in synergy to bring us myriad health benefits. Only in plants.

Michael Greger says:

> "The leading candidate class of compounds responsible for the protection against Alzheimer's are the phenolics, like flavones, and flavonones, and flavonols, which in many cases can rapidly cross the blood-brain barrier. There are more than 5,000 different types of flavonoids in the plants we eat. Research suggests that within minutes of biting into an apple, for example, these phytonutrients are already starting to light up our brain."

[See: http://nutritionfacts.org/video/phytochemicals-the-nutrition-facts-missing-from-the-label/]

There are a few phytos in the animals we eat – cows and sheeps and chooks are, after all, plantivores, not raptors. That said, there are pathetically few. On average, there're more than 60 times as many phytonutes in plants than in the animals that eat plants. Plants *are* phytonutrients. (In fact, 'phytonutrient' is a tautology: because only plants are food, all nutrients are phytonutrients.) Every mouthful of nutrient-free animal displaces more than 60 mouthfuls of nutrient-packed plants.

Anyone interested in learning more about the healing powers of plants should read Dr. Michael Greger's *How Not to Die: Discover the Foods Scientifically Proven to Prevent and Reverse Disease.*

Meating is a phytonutrient deficiency disease.

4. Nutrient density

When we come down to it, animals and junk are the exact opposite of food. They're overly endowed with bad stuff – especially fat-stored energy – and underendowed with nutrients. Animals and Junk are calorie-dense but nutrient-poor. Food, on the other hand, is calorie-lean and nutrient-hyper-dense. Animals and Junk lack appropriate nutrient density. Insulin resistance is just one of the ways junky, processed plants affect us in the same bad way as processed animals.

In the words of T. Colin Campbell: "There is no nutrient in animals that's not better supplied by plants."

Meating and Junking are nutrient-to-energy ratio imbalance diseases.

5. Plant proteins

Plant proteins differ from animal proteins in most beneficial ways. For example, plant proteins have lower amounts of the acidifying sulfur-containing amino acids, and lower amounts of leucine and methionine, the limitation of which has been shown to be life-extending. Plant proteins also don't cause the cross-reactivity problems that lead to auto-immune responses.

Meating isn't only a plant protein deficiency disease; it's an animal protein overdose disease.

5a. Glutamic acid

Glutamic acid is an amino acid found in many plants, and it has a strong independent blood pressure-lowering effect; independent meaning that plants in general lower BP, but glutamine can do it on its own. Animals have much lower glutamic acid levels; Meaters have higher BP.

6. Plant fats

Plant fats are different to animal fats both in their relative amounts in food and in their constitution. While Meaters get >30%, Planters get about 10% of their calories from fats, an ideal amount both for weight maintenance and peak performance. Same paleo diets are way more than 50% fat. The fats in whole plants tend to be unsaturated and anti-atherogenic, while those in processed animals and processed plants tend to be saturated, pro-inflammatory and pro-atherogenic.

Meating is a dose-dependent animal fat disease; a plant fat deficiency syndrome.

7. Carbohydrates

Other than the lactose in mothers' breast milk, and a tiny amount of stored glycogen in muscles, animals make no sugars at all. Glucose is the simple sugar that makes up both digestible starches and 'indigestible' fiber. Glucose is our most efficient fuel, though, in its absence, fats and proteins – even nucleic acids! – can be burned in an emergency situation.

As solar powered beings, we're adapted to eat liquid sunshine: sugar. Not table sugar. Not high fructose corn syrup. Sugar, as made by plants out of sunshine, water and our exhalations, then packaged with fiber and countless nutrients into… food.

Eating animals is a sugar-deficiency disease. The only healthy part of low-carb diets is the Planting.

8. Fiber

Fiber is fascinating stuff. I've been following the fiber story ever since 1974, when one of my heroes, Dr Dennis Burkitt gave a lecture in Cape Town titled "On Human Ordure." (As an English surgeon, I'm not sure he used the title 'Doctor.' In inverse snobbery, I suspect, surgeons in England tend to be called 'Mister.')

Burkitt and other physicians working in East Africa, like Hugh Trowell, noticed that constipation, diverticulosis and colorectal cancer weren't just rare among the predominantly plant-eating local population: they were absent. So too were the heart attacks, hypertension and strokes common in the West.

They put this down to the huge amounts of fiber in the traditional sub-Saharan African diet. Well, they were wrong… and they were right. Fiber itself may not be doing all the heavy lifting, so, when reductionists do experiments with fiber and nothing but the fiber, they sometimes fail to get good results. (This is why fiber substitutes like psyllium husks are a waste of time.) But…

When we use foods that are full of fiber then we get the results that Burkitt, Trowell et al got: a massive reduction in degenerative "diseases" across the board, particularly inflammatory bowel conditions.

Almost all Americans fail to meet the recommended daily fiber intake, including most vegans, who eat too much processed junk. 96% fail to eat adequate amounts of beans or greens. 99% don't eat enough grains.

There's zero fiber in animals, and precious little in junk. While Meating is a fiber-deficiency disease that causes a host of symptoms, from constipation to breast cancer, there are fiber-associated phytonutrients that are just as important as the fiber itself. One of them is:

9. Phytate ~ phytic acid

Discovered in 1903, phytates are a class of phosphorus-containing, saturated cyclic acid antioxidants found in all plant seeds: whole grains, beans, peas and lentils, nuts and seeds. They're what sprouting seeds feed on when they germinate, so you can imagine what wonderful nutrients they are – phyto-breast milk! Sprouts and micro-greens are intensely healthy.

Phytates have long been thought to be anti-nutrients because they were thought to lower our absorption of some minerals… but maybe we're looking at things the wrong way. Who says that lots of absorption is always a good thing? Unregulated heme iron absorption isn't good. Supplements are megadoses of micronutrients, and many of those shorten our lives. More isn't always better.

There are **mineral absorption enhancers** in plants, particularly in the allium family, that boost absorption, so if we're worried about our whole grain pasta inhibiting zinc or iron absorption, we can just add some onions or garlic, leeks or scallions to the tomato sauce. Oh, you do already? Great. Calamity averted.

(Someone once asked Winston Churchill to define the difference between a calamity and a catastrophe. He said: "If Clement Attlee fell into the Thames it would be a calamity. If someone fished him out again, that would be a catastrophe." He also said of Attlee that he was a modest man, who had much to be modest about, and that he was "a sheep in sheep's clothing." Some ill-feeling there, I think.)

But there wasn't a calamity anyway. The fear turned out to be fear of fear itself. The old anti-nutrient story about phytates was a canard based on ancient animal studies, now superseded by human data. Women who eat the most phytates have the best bone density – with higher calcium and phosphorus levels – so Planter phytate-eaters have the least osteoporosis.

To *not* eat phytonutrient-packed nuts and seeds, beans and grains every day is to eat our bones fragile. Late-life bone fractures are a consequence of lack of load-bearing exercise plus the eating disorder I've called Meating.

Besides lowering our risk of osteoporosis, phytates are powerful anti-cancer agents.

Do you remember how I said earlier (under Fiber) that there are phyto-nutrients that are bound to fiber that may be doing the heavy lifting on behalf of fiber (playing bellhop to fiber's concierge)? It's the phytate.

In Michael Greger's pithy words:

> "Dietary phytate, rather than fiber per se, might be **the most important variable governing the frequency of colon cancer,** as we know phytate is a **powerful inhibitor of the iron-mediated production of hydroxyl radicals**, a particularly dangerous type of free radical. So the standard American diet [Meating + Junking] may be a double whammy, the heme iron [a pro-oxidant or free radical producer] in muscle meat plus the lack of phytate in refined plant foods to extinguish the iron radicals."

[See: http://nutritionfacts.org/video/phytates-for-the-treatment-of-cancer/]

So, Burkitt and his colleagues were right to promote high fiber consumption, but maybe not for the fiber alone – we didn't know about phytate's marvelous anti-cancer properties back then. Diverticulosis and colorectal cancer are, indeed, fiber-deficiency conditions brought on by eating fiber-free animals and junk. Changing the magnification, we can say that Western "diseases" such as diverticulitis and colon cancer are also phytate-deficiency diseases.

Phytates are bound to fiber – no fiber, no phytates. Conversely, adding fiber to our diet doesn't add phytates. That's why Meater broscientists love to perform this following sleight of hand: fiber supplements don't prevent colon cancer (agreed, they don't, for the reason we now know – phytate deficiency); therefore eating plants doesn't prevent colon cancer. Gnur? No Planter has ever advocated eating isolated fiber as a proxy for Planting. Using it as one is a cheap shot. Planting drops our risk of inflammatory bowel symptoms like a put-ed shot.

The more animals we eat, the more cancer we get – not just bowel cancer. Cows double our risk. Chickens triple it. Beans and grains – all phytate-filled seeds – slice our risk like a knife through hot potatoes. (That's why the animal industry adds phytates to its dead products...)

Besides combatting cancer via antioxidation, phytates have multiple other anti-cancer mechanisms, beyond the scope of this discussion. Please just take it from me that these are powerful phytochemicals, and that we should eat whole plants every day to pack ourselves full of them (to phyte the good health phyte, daily).

(For more, see Dr. Greger's outstanding coverage in his book, *How Not to Die*, and in his online video "Phytates for Rehabilitating Cancer Cells.")

Also, high phytate intake → less diabetes + less heart "disease" + fewer kidney stones.

Plus phytates put their mineral-grabbing powers to use on heavy metals such as lead and cadmium, so that Planters could eat more mercury [it doesn't happen], and still have lower mercury blood levels than Meaters. Grain- and bean-eating lowers our risk of heavy metal toxicity! Double!!

I did an online search for a definition of 'vitamin' and I got "any of a group of organic compounds which are essential for normal growth and nutrition and are required in small quantities in the diet because they cannot be synthesized by the body."

Well, we need it and we can't make it, so phytic acid qualifies as a vitamin or essential-to-eat, unnecessary-to-make-because-ubiquitous-in-food nutrient, and may eventually make its way into the accepted canon, which presently numbers a last-supper-ish 13. (Were there waiters? No need, I guess, with such a simple meal.)

Historically, vitamins have come and gone, reflecting our current knowledge of physiology. For a while, laetrile – isolated from apricot pips – was called vitamin B_{17}. It's since been demoted. Sad, really; tasting glory, then blithely discarded. (As I'll mention later, there are two other phyto-candidates for vitaminhood (vitamancy would be too confusing.))

Meating and Junking are potentially lethal phytate vitamin-deficiency diseases.

10. Gut flora
The old view of 'indigestible' fiber or 'roughage' is that it's supposed to be the cellulose part of plants that we can't digest, and it's beneficial because it bulks out our stools, aids peristalsis, binds up cholesterol/bile acids and estrogens and flushes them out, while it itself remains undigested… a kind of poop catalyst.

As we now know, "we" *can* digest fiber. By "we" I mean, we humans working in tandem with the trillions of gut bacteria who live within us, particularly in our bowels, and who greatly outnumber our human cells.

Our gut flora digests fiber. They thrive on fiber. They ferment it and produce wonderful products, of use to them and to us. We feed them and they feed us.

I find our gut flora (and our enteric (gut) nervous system) fascinating. We can change our gut flora, depending on what we feed them. This is absolutely essential to understand:

We should think of our gut flora as making up a separate anatomical organ. That's how important they are to digestion and metabolism.

Different populations of bacteria take up residence in our guts depending on what we feed them.

Planters and Meaters have different gut flora: you won't see this on an anatomical chart or in a textbook, but **Planters and Meaters have different digestive tracts**. Different bodies! Meating changes our bodies by deranging our gut flora. Feeding our gut flora decomposing animals actively selects for gut flora that decompose dead animals. We live in harmony with our gut flora when we're Planters.

Within our gut flora, some species are definitely healthier than others. Phytonutrients such as the polyphenols found in green tea, in fruits like apples and grapes, and in the vinegars made from them encourage *Prevotella* species such as *Faecalibacterium prausnitzii* to flourish, while discouraging *Bacteroides* species (which is good, because the latter are associated with increased immune response and more inflammation.) Animals do the exact opposite.

If instead of feeding our intestinal bacteria with fiber to ferment, we feed them animal proteins to rot, we shouldn't be surprised when we get different, sulfur-emitting results. Fermentation is beneficial; putrefaction by baleful species such as *Bilophila wadsworthia* is decidedly not.

Meating is a gut flora-deranging disease.

For more, see The Eatiology of Obesity #15: Enterotypes, in Part 1C: Eatiology

11. Propionate

When we feed our friendly gut bacteria on the fiber they love, they digest it for us and make a substance called propionate, which we absorb through our gut walls into our bloodstream. It turns out that fiber is digestible by humans – we just have to change our definition of human. We need to rewrite the human anatomy texts to include a virtual digestive organ known as our gut flora. It doesn't matter if it doesn't appear in *Grey's Anatomy*; it appears in us and has always done so. We're slowly getting wise to its/their existence.

Propionate slows the synthesis of cholesterol. (Here's another double whammy for Meaters, who get the negative of too much cholesterol to begin with, plus the lack of the positive propionate effect from plants.) Propionate also slows down our stomach emptying and creates a feeling of satiety, which combines in a **hypophagic effect**. Hypo = less, and phagic = eating. The propionate from bacteria-digested fiber makes us eat less.

The hypophagic effect of propionate, the effects of healthy *Bacteroides* gut flora species, the lower energy density (and higher nutrient density) of plants, the avoidance of animal-borne obesogenic viruses and chemical obesogens, the bulkiness of fiber that triggers pressure sensors in our intestinal walls signaling fullness, and the thermogenic effect (see later) and increased brown fat deposition (later), both of which speed up Planters' metabolisms, leading to more calories being expended as heat, are multiple mechanisms which combine to make Planters the only group of eaters to have ideal body weight (BMI < 25).

As a group, Planters are the slenderest people in the world. This isn't wishful thinking; it's demonstrated scientific fact. (We've seen some of the great Adventist studies, comparing different dietstyles' effects on obesity, diabetes, hypertension and heart "disease". Each of these conditions gets worse, dose-dependently, with increased animal consumption.)

While Meaters and Junkers feel the need to take probiotics to promote a healthy gut flora, Planters don't. Planters use prebiotics. In other words, Planters just eat food. Planting feeds our gut flora their meal of choice – fiber – and that encourages the healthiest possible gut flora to thrive. Eating fiber encourages fiber-eating bacteria, who in turn feed us propionate, with its amazing anti-obesity qualities. Eat plants… they will come.

Fiber-depleted Meating and Junking are propionate deficiency diseases.

12. Lignans

Lignans are a class of anti-carcinogenic phytonutrients found in seeds and nuts, particularly flax seeds and walnuts. Actually, there are zero lignans in flax: our gut flora makes them for us out of their lignan precursors in nuts and seeds.

Lignans are phytoestrogens that help prevent breast and prostate cancer in particular. Meaters' gut flora isn't purpose-built for making lignans. Meaters' gut flora, lacking in fiber and disturbed by sulfur, have adapted to eating dead animals. That's why Meaters become so farty when eating beans – the wrong bacteria for digesting beans, or nuts and seeds. So, it's a double whammy for Meaters – more carcinogens in what we eat when we Meat, and fewer of the cancer-fighters served up on Planters' plates.

Meating is a lignan-deficiency disease.

13. Butyrate

Butyrate is yet another substance that our gut bacteria make for us, also out of fiber, like propionate. Butyrate is a short chain fatty acid with anti-inflammatory and anti-cancer properties.

Butyrate is what fuels the cells that make up our colon walls. We and our bacteria are partners in dining: we feed each other… as long as we don't eat animals. Eating animals encourages the wrong species of bacteria to take over. There's no possible way for bacteria to make butyrate both out of carbohydrate and out of animals – there's zero carbohydrate in animals. We're sugar-powered sweeties, not ghouls.

The more fiber we eat, the more butyrate-producing bacteria there are in our colons. We don't change our genes by eating fiber, but epigenetic changes take place so that the more bacteria there are, the more butyrate-producing genes get switched on. Fiber eating upregulates the genes for butyrate production.

Butyrate is a large part of the reason why Planters get so much less colon cancer and ulcerative colitis than Meaters; the presence of butyrate, and the absence of the cytotoxic gas, hydrogen sulfide, that our gut bacteria produce from animal proteins.

(If something we eat induces our gut flora to make an oxidative, DNA-damaging cell poison out of it, should we call it food?)

Propionate, lignans and butyrate are three very large gifts our good bacteria give us; gifts that Meaters spurn, their bacteria not having been given the gift of fiber. Or, if Meaters do eat fiber, the animals they've eaten have encouraged animal-eating gut bacteria, which are less able to produce propionate or butyrate. Meating not only introduces obesogenic, inflammatory, and carcinogenic agents, but Meaters lose out on the wondrous anti-obesity, anti-inflammatory and anti-cancer agents produced by plant-fed bacteria.

Meating is a (sulfur overdose and) butyrate deficiency disease.

14. Minerals

Minerals are powdered rocks. They're the inorganic part of soil, from where they're incorporated into plants as they grow. Minerals need to be taken up by plants to become bioavailable at appropriate concentrations. Taking a rock and using a grater to sprinkle some stone particles into our food, as if we're cows at a salt lick, may work too well. Plants are the kitchen workers who prepare minerals for the dining pleasure of animals… like us humans. We don't need to pass minerals through animals before ingesting them. Other animals get their minerals from plants. So should we.

In some cases, Meating is a mineral deficiency disease. In others, Meating is a mineral overdose disease. Planters absorb minerals in Goldilocks amounts: not too many, not too few, right in the middle in the sweet spot, with phytonutrients that limit or boost absorption, depending on how much we need.

More isn't better. As we saw above, plant copper, plant iron and plant phosphorus are all better regulated than their animal counterparts, which are prone to overload, setting us up for kidney failure and dementia. On the other hand, plant calcium is far better absorbed than animal.

Junking and Meating are mineral-inefficiency diseases.

15. Magnesium

Unsurprisingly, animal eaters are often deficient in magnesium, the ion at the heart of the chlorin ring in chlorophyll. (Not chlorine; chlorin.) The majority of Americans don't meet the recommended minimum intake.

The following list shows the first of 311 online pages of magnesium-containing foods and non-foods adapted from the USDA's National Nutrient Database for Standard Reference Release 27. You'll notice that no non-foods make it onto the page. There's nothing but nuts, seeds, beans and grains… and molasses, though I think non-bears would find a cup of molasses hard to swallow.

Food is where we find magnesium. The only two animal sources to crack the top 100 are conch at #76 and (enhanced!) turkey at #80. So, one rare sea animal, and one animal + supplement.

NDB_No	Description	Weight(g)	Measure	Magnesium, Mg (mg) Per Measure
20060	Rice bran, crude	118	1.0 cup	922
19304	Molasses	337	1.0 cup	816
12014	Seeds, pumpkin and squash seed kernels, dried	129	1.0 cup	764
16078	Mothbeans, mature seeds, raw	196	1.0 cup	747
12007	Seeds, cottonseed flour, partially defatted (glandless)	94	1.0 cup	678
12160	Seeds, cottonseed kernels, roasted (glandless)	149	1.0 cup	656
12016	Seeds, pumpkin and squash seed kernels, roasted, without salt	118	1.0 cup	649
12516	Seeds, pumpkin and squash seed kernels, roasted, with salt added	118	1.0 cup	649
16067	Hyacinth beans, mature seeds, raw	210	1.0 cup	594
16133	Yardlong beans, mature seeds, raw	167	1.0 cup	564
12174	Seeds, watermelon seed kernels, dried	108	1.0 cup	556
16060	Cowpeas, catjang, mature seeds, raw	167	1.0 cup	556
16083	Mungo beans, mature seeds, raw	207	1.0 cup	553
16108	Soybeans, mature seeds, raw	186	1.0 cup	521
12201	Seeds, sesame seed kernels, dried (decorticated)	150	1.0 cup	518
43299	Soybean, curd cheese	225	1.0 cup	513
12023	Seeds, sesame seeds, whole, dried	144	1.0 cup	505
12078	Nuts, brazilnuts, dried, unblanched	133	1.0 cup	500
20001	Amaranth grain, uncooked	193	1.0 cup	479
12529	Seeds, sesame seed kernels, toasted, with salt added (decorticated)	128	1.0 cup	443
12029	Seeds, sesame seed kernels, toasted, without salt added (decorticated)	128	1.0 cup	443
16047	Beans, yellow, mature seeds, raw	196	1.0 cup	435
12065	Nuts, almonds, oil roasted, without salt added	157	1.0 cup	430
12565	Nuts, almonds, oil roasted, with salt added	157	1.0 cup	430
12665	Nuts, almonds, oil roasted, lightly salted	157	1.0 cup	430

National Nutrient Database for Standard Reference Release 27: Magnesium

Why's magnesium important? Magnesium is one of the minerals that maintain our bodies' electrical systems. Our heartbeats are controlled by electrical impulses, and magnesium is our drummer (Hi, Debs. Hi, Gary.) It's the positive ion that keeps the rhythm going. Arrhythmias result from magnesium deficiency (and bass players).

Being low in magnesium sets us up for Sudden Cardiac Death, which accounts for more than half of all deaths from our #1 killer, heart "disease".

Death via SCD is the first symptom, or warning, the majority of heart attack victims get of their heart "disease". 'Healthy' one moment; dead the next. Only about 2% of Americans meet their daily requirement of magnesium. Seeing as the top sources of magnesium are seeds, nuts and grains, I'll leave it to you to work out who makes up the bulk of the 2% of adequate mag-eaters. (I believe that vegans now make up about 2% of the population, but there may be many Junkers within the vegan ranks.)

Just an ounce (28g) of seeds or nuts a day, added to the crappy SAD diet could extend many tens of thousands of American lives each year.

Meating and Junking are magnesium deficiency diseases. Sudden Cardiac Death is often a first symptom of Meating with the unfortunate character flaw of being a 'last word freak.'

16. Calcium

For all that the dairy industries of the world tell us otherwise, their products aren't a particularly good source of calcium. (They're a pretty good source of pus though, in case we think we're running low?)

Countries that have the highest dairy consumption suffer from the highest rates of osteoporosis. (Yes, we'll correlate away, my friends – we know the difference between correlation and causation, and there's plenty of other evidence to back the epidemiology.) The Asians who have the good fortune to be lactose intolerant and who consume no dairy products at all have no osteoporosis. (Those who do, do.) Osteoporosis can be as much or more a consequence of lack of load-bearing exercise than lack of calcium or magnesium or phosphorus or boron. It's the result of a sedentary lifestyle coupled with the eating of animals. Having enough vitamin D is also important, so we should all bear our loads outdoors when we can.

Phyto-calcium is absorbed half again as well as animal milk and cheese calcium, without the side order of Parkinson's.

Meating is a calcium-deficient diet; but junk "food" veganism can be too – we need to eat our whole greens and beans, dear peeps, every day!

17. Potassium

Potassium is another mineral Meaters struggle to get enough of. Showing why, below, is the first page of the National Nutrient Database for Standard Reference Release 27, for potassium per 100g.

It looks like the word 'herb' isn't in the USDA's lexicon. I tend to use 'herb' for plant leaves and 'spice' for all the other parts. I wouldn't call tarragon a spice. But, hey, it took a court case to change tomatoes from fruits into vegetables, so I may have missed the Supreme Court's spice ruling.

Upping one's potassium levels seriously reduces one's risk of stroke, much the same way increased magnesium intake seriously cuts one's risk of arrhythmia and heart attack. 98% of Americans are deficient in potassium; meaning, basically, that all Meaters are potassium-deficient and at risk of stroke. Well, we knew that anyway, because stroke is the #4 cause of death, after heart "disease", cancer and lung "disease".

The best way to avoid stroke is to stop Meating and go on a high-potassium Planter diet, with plenty of beans and leafy green veggies. Sun-dried tomatoes and sweet peppers are great sources.

NDB_No	Description	Potassium, K (mg) Value Per 100g
18373	Leavening agents, cream of tartar	16,500.00
18371	Leavening agents, baking powder, low-sodium	10,100.00
11625	Parsley, freeze-dried	6,300.00
14353	Tea, instant, unsweetened, powder, decaffeinated	6,040.00
14366	Tea, instant, unsweetened, powder	6,040.00
2008	Spices, chervil, dried	4,740.00
2012	Spices, coriander leaf, dried	4,466.00
14203	Coffee, instant, regular, powder, half the caffeine	3,535.00
14214	Coffee, instant, regular, powder	3,535.00
14218	Coffee, instant, decaffeinated, powder	3,501.00
11432	Radishes, oriental, dried	3,494.00
14368	Tea, instant, unsweetened, lemon-flavored, powder	3,453.00
11955	Tomatoes, sun-dried	3,427.00
14222	Coffee, instant, with chicory, powder	3,395.00
2017	Spices, dill weed, dried	3,308.00
11634	Peppers, sweet, green, freeze-dried	3,170.00
11931	Peppers, sweet, red, freeze-dried	3,170.00
14409	Beverages, Orange-flavor drink, breakfast type, low calorie, powder	3,132.00
16425	Soy sauce, reduced sodium, made from hydrolyzed vegetable protein	3,098.00
2041	Spices, tarragon, dried	3,020.00
11615	Chives, freeze-dried	2,960.00
31019	Seaweed, Canadian Cultivated EMI-TSUNOMATA, dry	2,944.00
14196	Cocoa mix, no sugar added, powder	2,702.00
14538	Beverages, Cocoa mix, low calorie, powder, with added calcium, phosp	2,702.00
2029	Spices, parsley, dried	2,683.00

National Nutrient Database for Standard Reference Release 27: Potassium

Meating is a potassium deficiency disease.

18. Iodine

Getting enough iodine can be a problem for all of us, Meaters and Planters alike. For optimal health, we need to get adequate iodine, which is a component of thyroid hormones, otherwise we may get a thyroid growth called a goiter. Not pretty.

According to the NIH, under Food Sources, at https://ods.od.nih.gov/factsheets/Iodine-HealthProfessional/: "Seaweed (such as kelp, nori, kombu, and wakame) is one of the best food sources of iodine, but it is highly variable in its content... Other good sources include seafood, dairy products (partly due to the use of iodine feed supplements and iodophor sanitizing agents in the dairy industry, grain products, and eggs. Dairy products, especially milk, and grain products are the major contributors of iodine to the American diet."

The iodine in commercial dairy products is partly from supplements; also partly from iodine contamination with disinfectants used in milk tanks and on often-swollen, mastitic cow udders. (More than 15% of cows in the US have mastitis, a staph infection, so the odds of staph in milk tanks is 100%.) I think I'll pass. And I think I'll skip the seafood [oxymoron alert], because of the bonus heavy metals; and the eggs because of the free cholesterol (a single yolk putting us over our 'safe' daily upper limit). (Wouldn't it be nice if Kevin Bacon, egg tout for the American Egg Board, actually knew something about nutrition?) "Food is a package deal," so iodine is best found in sea vegetables (but not hijiki/hiziki because of arsenic contamination, and not kelp, because it contains too much iodine.)

Curiously, the USDA's National Nutrient Database for Standard Reference Release 27 doesn't list iodine as a nutrient. Which puzzles me, because the list is fairly comprehensive. For example, they do list alcohol, caffeine and theobromine, so boozehounds, Java junkies and chocoholics can all do a quick search to get the biggest bangs for their bucks. But no iodine…

And my other go-to source for nutrient numbers, SELFNutritionData at http://nutritiondata.self.com, is similarly reticent. Type in 'kelp' (a single gram of which, according to the NIH, provides between 11% and 1,989% (!!) of one's DV (daily value)), and we get the news that kelp is high in sodium, but not a single word about iodine. Using their 'nutrient search' tool also comes up empty. It looks like they get their info from the USDA database.

(There may be a quite logical explanation for this iodine coyness, one that's known to non-amateur nutrition enthusiasts such as myself: a kind of shibboleth, which allows outsiders to be slaughtered for mispronouncing the word. I'd love to know… Perhaps iodine is too dangerous to make recommendations about? The variation in kelp above is certainly concerning: 11 to 1,989 is an astonishing range of almost three orders of magnitude. My guess is that iodine is too variable in its sources to make concrete dietary intake recommendations.)

Iodine is tricky, so Planters, Junkers and Meaters – all of us, except the prana-sustained breatharians – are all at risk of iodine-deficiency, so we need to give it some thought.

Sidebar: A quick rant about the National Nutrient Database
The USDA's nutrition database is horribly flawed. It lists nutrients in two searchable ways – either by hundred gram portions or by household, in which they choose measures which they think are suitable, such as cups of

grains or kilo slabs of cow's ribs. This is absolute craziness. None of us has a daily intake requirement for weights and measures of food – we don't need to eat 2 cups of this or a thousand grams of that.

What we do each have is an energy requirement of (very) roughly 2000 - 2500 calories per day; an energy requirement that should be divided up among all the nutrients we need to eat each day. We need to get at least 100% of all our nutrients every day, or on average over a period of time, while staying within our calorie budget. What point is there in getting 100% of our nutrients, if it takes 150% of our energy requirement to get there? Listing nutrients by weight or household doesn't help with this.

All nutrients should be listed by multiples of calories, not by weight! This is an absolute fundamental principle of studying food, Nutrition 101, and the USDA gets it wrong.

Why?

Because the USDA caters to animal agriculture. Listing nutrients by weight instead of calories makes animals look better and plants look worse. Why? Because animals are energy-dense and nutrient-poor, while plants are nutrient-dense and energy-sparse. Meating and Junking provide at least three times as much fat as Planting, and fat itself provides 2.25 times as much energy per gram as the other macronutrients. (Fat, 9 calories per gram; alcohol, 7; protein and carbs, 4.)

Planters get more of all nutrients while eating fewer calories. This is the concept of nutrient density, popularized by Dr. Joel Fuhrman and others.

All that data… and the USDA hasn't presented it in a way that makes meaningful comparisons between plants, junk and animals possible. It's not quite useless, but it should be a lot better. The USDA should be ashamed of themselves for their incompetence or deviousness, whichever it is.

The Meater USDA as a whole, and their Meater dietary guidelines committees in particular, are probably the single major reason why the USA became the fattest population ever to exist. Them, and the inventors of HFCS. (Note: I believe we've recently lost this dubious #1 distinction… to populations who eat just like us, only more so.)

Kudos to SELFNutritionData for allowing us to search their nutrient database the right way: by 200 calorie servings.

19. Nitrates

When dealing with nitrites earlier, I went into the importance of nitrates for vascular health. While nitrites abound naturally in animals and also in preservatives used in animals, animals are spectacularly poor sources of nitrates. Leafy green vegetables are nitrate bonanzas.

When we're Meaters, the closest some of us come to this beneficial form of nitrogen may be from fertilizer residues or from the nitroglycerine tablet we suck on desperately, to counteract the crushing cardiac pain known as angina (a symptom of Meating).

Meating is a nitrate deficiency disease.

20. Phytoestrogens

This one's dead easy. Phytoestrogens are beneficial endocrine disruptors in plants that block out the effect of animal estrogens and environmental estrogen disruptors that bioaccumulate in animals, lowering our risk of estrogenic cancers. There aren't any in animals.

Meating is a phytoestrogen deficiency disease.

21. Vitamins

As I mentioned when discussing the miracle of chlorophyll, all the vitamins are made by plants, except for two, one of which is made by bacteria (B_{12}), and one (D) by the action of sunlight on animal skin, us being the animals in question.

This being the case, Meating is a vitamin deficiency disease, unless accompanied by liberal doses of Planting.

22. Vitamin A

Vitamin A supplements and beta-carotene supplements shorten our lives. Planters have higher levels of A than Meaters. Meaters who try to address their deficiency shouldn't do it by Junking – taking supplements – but by Planting.

Meaters should also not get their A from cod liver oil, even if it is the top-ranked source in the USDA database, below.

Supplements are dangerous non-foods and we shouldn't eat them… except for cobalamin (B_{12}).

USDA National Nutrient Database for Standard ReferenceRelease 27

Nutrients: Vitamin A, IU (IU)

Food Subset: All Foods
Ordered by: Nutrient Content
Measured by: 100 g
Report Run at: February 01, 2015 12:21 EST

NDB_No	Description
04589	Fish oil, cod liver
23425	Beef, New Zealand, imported, liver, raw
11931	Peppers, sweet, red, freeze-dried
17203	Veal, variety meats and by-products, liver, cooked, braised
23424	Beef, New Zealand, imported, liver, cooked, boiled
11683	Carrot, dehydrated
11615	Chives, freeze-dried

National Nutrient Database for Standard Reference Release 27: Vitamin A

23. Folate (Vitamin B₉)

Folate is another of the phytonutrients in which Meaters tend to be deficient. They're best obtained from beans and green foliage.

While plant folate is beneficial, folic acid in supplements is harmful. Folate is cancer-protective; synthetic folic acid, carcinogenic.

Meating is a folate deficiency disease.

24. B vitamins (thiamin, riboflavin, niacin, pyridoxine, folate et al)

In general, Planters have higher levels of the B vitamins than Meaters, always supposing we take our B_{12}.

As mentioned in section 1, homocysteine is an intermediary metabolite between two other sulfur-containing amino acids, methionine and cysteine. I went to some length describing how much more of these amino acids there is in animals, and also how damaging they can be to our health. For example, methionine restriction is an acknowledge method of slowing down the aging process.

Elevated levels of homocysteine are associated with blood clots, heart attacks and strokes; also with cognitive decline and Alzheimer's.

Three of the B vitamins are crucial for maintaining brain health by detoxifying homocysteine. It looks like this:

B_6 + B_9 + B_{12} → lower concentration of homocysteine → less cognitive decline or Alzheimer's.

A shortage of any of these three B vitamins can cause hyperhomocysteinemia (a fancy way of saying elevated homocysteine levels), so it's important to keep all three high. As borne out by population studies, Planters who keep topped up with B_{12} have better levels of the other two Bs and consequently better brain health than Meaters, but Planters who neglect B_{12} can end up with stiffened, enflamed arteries just like Meaters, and cognitive decline.

Most people get enough pyridoxine (B_6), so for Meaters, the limiting B vitamin for detoxing homocysteine is folate (B_9), found mainly in green leafies and beans.

(Only 4% of Americans meet the pathetically low suggested daily intake levels for either leafy greens or beans, which puts 96% of the population at risk for brain damage via homocysteine. I guess that makes dementia-by-malnutrition 'normal.')

Other Meater factors that worsen our risk for Alzheimer's include inflammation via arachidonic acid, amyloidosis via animal proteins, heme iron, increased copper and aluminum toxicity, and cardiogenic dementia, via cholesterol-induced atherosclerosis.

25. Beta- and the carotenes
No, not a 60s-era pop band from Liverpool. Beta-carotene is just the best-known of more than 500 carotene phytonutrients. All of them play a role, not just one, and they work synergistically… the total being immeasurably greater than the sum of the parts.

Beta-carotene supplements are life-shortening. They're not food and we shouldn't eat them.

26. Vitamin C
While vitamin C is a fabulous general-purpose antioxidant, it plays a special role in boosting iron absorption from plants. (We've already seen that we can't regulate intake of heme iron from animal blood.) Our bodies aren't dumb. Iron creates lots of free radicals, so how better to manage iron intake than to have the antioxidant responsible for defusing the iron be the one who's working the door for crowd control, deciding who and how many get in?

In plants, the bomb and the bomb disposal expert come packaged together in one food. With animals, we keep chucking bombs into the crowd, without a bomb techy anywhere in sight.

Take a look below at page 1 of old standby, the USDA's nutrient database page for vitamin C. There's not much there in the way of real food, but I think you get the drift. Animals need not apply.

Besides being a disease of heme iron toxicity, Meating is a vitamin C deficiency disease.

USDA National Nutrient Database for Standard ReferenceRelease 27

Nutrients: Vitamin C, total ascorbic acid (mg)

Food Subset: All Foods
Ordered by: Nutrient Content
Measured by: 100 g
Report Run at: February 01, 2015 12:05 EST

NDB_No	Description
14409	Beverages, Orange-flavor drink, breakfast type, low calorie, powder
43345	Fruit-flavored drink, powder, with high vitamin C with other added vitamins, low calorie
11634	Peppers, sweet, green, freeze-dried
11931	Peppers, sweet, red, freeze-dried
09001	Acerola, (west indian cherry), raw
09002	Acerola juice, raw
11615	Chives, freeze-dried
02012	Spices, coriander leaf, dried
42055	Fruit-flavored drink, dry powdered mix, low calorie, with aspartame
19703	Gelatin desserts, dry mix, reduced calorie, with aspartame, added phosphorus, potassium, sodium, vitamin C
25016	Formulated bar, MARS SNACKFOOD US, SNICKERS MARATHON Energy Bar, all flavors
35203	Rose Hips, wild (Northern Plains Indians)
25003	Snacks, candy rolls, yogurt-covered, fruit flavored with high vitamin C
43544	Babyfood, cereal, rice with pears and apple, dry, instant
14424	Orange-flavor drink, breakfast type, with pulp, frozen concentrate
11670	Peppers, hot chili, green, raw
08504	Cereals ready-to-eat, RALSTON Enriched Wheat Bran flakes
14407	Orange-flavor drink, breakfast type, powder
09139	Guavas, common, raw
08028	Cereals ready-to-eat, KELLOGG, KELLOGG'S ALL-BRAN COMPLETE Wheat Flakes
08058	Cereals ready-to-eat, KELLOGG, KELLOGG'S PRODUCT 19
08077	Cereals ready-to-eat, GENERAL MILLS, Whole Grain TOTAL
16262	SILK Hazelnut Creamer
14426	Orange drink, breakfast type, with juice and pulp, frozen concentrate
11951	Peppers, sweet, yellow, raw
09165	Litchis, dried
09083	Currants, european black, raw
25043	Snacks, candy bits, yogurt covered with vitamin C

National Nutrient Database for Standard Reference Release 27: Vitamin C

27. Vitamin E

On the next page is the USDA on antioxidant vitamin E. Junk tops the list in the form of processed vegetable oils and cereals, but the point is: Plants only. Sunflower seeds are the best whole-food source. Nuts like almonds, hazelnuts or filberts are also excellent. Other good sources are green leafies and whole grains.

Nuts and seeds, because of their high vitamin E content, are protective against asthma, slashing risk in half.

Meating is a vitamin E deficiency disease.

NDB_No	Description
04038	Oil, wheat germ
08504	Cereals ready-to-eat, RALSTON Enriched Wheat Bran flakes
08590	Cereals ready-to-eat, KASHI HEART TO HEART, Warm Cinnamon
08387	Cereals ready-to-eat, KASHI HEART TO HEART, Honey Toasted Oat
14047	Beverages, UNILEVER, SLIMFAST Shake Mix, powder, 3-2-1 Plan
14055	Beverages, UNILEVER, SLIMFAST Shake Mix, high protein, powder, 3-2-1 Plan
04532	Oil, hazelnut
08028	Cereals ready-to-eat, KELLOGG, KELLOGG'S ALL-BRAN COMPLETE Wheat Flakes
08058	Cereals ready-to-eat, KELLOGG, KELLOGG'S PRODUCT 19
08077	Cereals ready-to-eat, GENERAL MILLS, Whole Grain TOTAL
08610	Cereals ready-to-eat, KASHI Honey Sunshine
16155	Peanut butter, smooth, vitamin and mineral fortified
16156	Peanut butter, chunky, vitamin and mineral fortified
08611	Cereals ready-to-eat, KELLOGG's FIBERPLUS Cinnamon Oat Crunch
04060	Oil, sunflower, linoleic (less than 60%)
04506	Oil, sunflower, linoleic, (approx. 65%)
04545	Oil, sunflower, linoleic, (partially hydrogenated)
04584	Oil, sunflower, high oleic (70% and over)
04642	Oil, industrial, mid-oleic, sunflower
04529	Oil, almond
02009	Spices, chili powder
04687	Margarine-like spread, BENECOL Light Spread
12038	Seeds, sunflower seed kernels, oil roasted, without salt
12538	Seeds, sunflower seed kernels, oil roasted, with salt added
35232	Wocas, dried seeds, Oregon, yellow pond lily (Klamath)
04502	Oil, cottonseed, salad or cooking
04702	Oil, industrial, cottonseed, fully hydrogenated
12036	Seeds, sunflower seed kernels, dried

National Nutrient Database for Standard Reference Release 27: Vitamin E

28. Vitamin K

Herbs (and other, larger) green leafy vegetables are where K is found.

In "Plant vs. Cow Calcium ," Michael Greger calls vitamin K a "bone health superstar." Higher vitamin K levels are yet another reason besides superior calcium absorption from plants, decreased acidosis from plants, decreased phosphorus levels from Planting and increased levels of potassium and magnesium that Planters have better bone health than Meaters: reduced risk of bone fracture and osteoporosis.

Meating is a vitamin K deficiency disease.

NDB_No	Description
02003	Spices, basil, dried
02038	Spices, sage, ground
02042	Spices, thyme, dried
11297	Parsley, fresh
02012	Spices, coriander leaf, dried
02029	Spices, parsley, dried
11003	Amaranth leaves, raw
11236	Kale, frozen, cooked, boiled, drained, without salt
11791	Kale, frozen, cooked, boiled, drained, with salt
11147	Chard, swiss, raw
11234	Kale, cooked, boiled, drained, without salt
02034	Spices, poultry seasoning
11207	Dandelion greens, raw
11233	Kale, raw
11164	Collards, frozen, chopped, cooked, boiled, drained, without salt
11769	Collards, frozen, chopped, cooked, boiled, drained, with salt
02023	Spices, marjoram, dried
02027	Spices, oregano, dried
11271	Mustard greens, cooked, boiled, drained, without salt
11799	Mustard greens, cooked, boiled, drained, with salt
11208	Dandelion greens, cooked, boiled, drained, without salt
11203	Cress, garden, raw
11464	Spinach, frozen, chopped or leaf, cooked, boiled, drained, without salt
11856	Spinach, frozen, chopped or leaf, cooked, boiled, drained, with salt
11575	Turnip greens, frozen, cooked, boiled, drained, without salt
11892	Turnip greens, frozen, cooked, boiled, drained, with salt
35205	Stinging Nettles, blanched (Northern Plains Indians)
11245	Lambsquarters, cooked, boiled, drained, without salt

National Nutrient Database for Standard Reference Release 27: Vitamin K

29. Ergothioneine

Ergothioneine is the first of the two phytochemicals I mentioned earlier that could qualify as a new vitamin. I bent the rules slightly though. Ergothioneine isn't a phytonutrient; it's a myconutrient, found in fungi like white button mushrooms, and it's also made by bacteria in the soil, just like B_{12}. There's definitely none in animals.

We need ergothioneine in small amounts and we can't make it: that makes it a nutrient essential for us to eat. A mushroom a week probably does the trick.

What does it do for us? It's an amino acid that's a potent antioxidant and cytoprotectant – it protects our cells from DNA damage, even inside our cell nuclei and mitochondria, which are particularly full of free radicals because they're our little cellular nuclear reactors.

According to Michael Greger:

> "Ergothioneine concentrates in parts of our body where there's lots of oxidative stress—the lens of our eye and the liver, as well as sensitive areas such as bone marrow and seminal fluid."

[See: http://nutritionfacts.org/video/ergothioneine-a-new-vitamin/]

Although most people haven't heard of this amazing quasi-vitamin, Meating is an ergothioneine deficiency disease.

30. Salicylic acid

Well, I didn't keep the suspense going for long: salicylic acid, the active ingredient in aspirin, is another phytonutrient that should probably also be classed as a vitamin. We need it in tiny quantities and we can't make it: ergo, vitamin. Originally isolated from willow tree bark, salicylic acid is present in small amounts virtually throughout the plant kingdom.

Considering that cardiologists often prescribe a baby aspirin a day to patients with heart "disease" to prevent blood clots and heart attacks, wouldn't it be easier to stop the Meating that causes the heart attacks and start Planting, which contains the doctor's remedy already? Can the salicylic acid (that's naturally in plants) be another reason why Planters have so much less heart "disease" than Meaters?

Yes, it can.

Meating is an aspirin-deficiency disease, not a statin-deficiency disease.

31. Neurotransmitters, part 1: serotonin

Neurotransmitters are the chemicals that make nerves work. When nerves transmit information as electrical impulses, neurotransmitters are chemicals which are released into synaptic clefts between nerve cells, or neurons, and they activate other nerve cells, or muscles or glands.

Serotonin, dopamine, melatonin and adrenaline (epinephrine) are all neurotransmitters… and they're made by plants! Of course, plants, not having nervous systems, use these chemicals for other purposes. It's a bit speciesist of us to call them neurotransmitters when their creators have been using them for billions of years for protection and flowering etc. They only become neurotransmitters when they're in Johnny-come-lately animals such as ourselves.

Serotonin is known as the "happiness hormone." A shortage of serotonin in our brains causes depression. There's a class of anti-depression drugs known as SSRIs (selective serotonin reuptake inhibitors), a very lucrative class of drugs which don't work very well and have serious (side-) effects. They supposedly work by preventing serotonin's reabsorption after release, making it persist longer, but placebos have been shown to work just as well, and placebos do squat to serotonin absorption.

Another way of boosting brain serotonin (besides preventing reabsorption) is to put more of it into our brains. But serotonin doesn't cross the blood-brain barrier, so eating plants for their serotonin doesn't work. Happily, a precursor of serotonin, the amino acid tryptophan, does get into the brain, allowing us to make more serotonin.

Plant tryptophan is particularly beneficial. Michael Greger lists "plantains, pineapples, bananas, kiwis, plums, and tomatoes" as excellent sources. There's also some tryptophan in animals, but there are so many other more aggressive amino acids in animals that animal tryptophan loses out in the competition for receptor sites.

[See: http://nutritionfacts.org/video/human-neurotransmitters-in-plants/]

Planting is the best frontline remedy for depression. Meating is a depressing serotonin-deficiency disease. Prozac and zoloft and tryptophan supplements aren't food, and we shouldn't eat them.

And absolutely no one should have brain stimulants like Ritalin inflicted upon them. We should just make our kids food, dear hearts. And exercise.

32. Neurotransmitters, part 2: dopamine

If serotonin is the "happiness hormone," dopamine is the "pleasure hormone." It's released, for example, during orgasm, lighting up the 'pleasure center' of our brains.

Here's what Michael Greger has to say about dopamine and Parkinson's:

> "At its root, Parkinson's is a dopamine deficiency disease, because of a die-off of dopamine-generating cells in the brain. These cells make dopamine from L-DOPA derived from an amino acid in our diet [L-tyrosine], but just like we saw with the serotonin story, the

consumption of animal products blocks the transport of L-DOPA into the brain, crowding it out."

[See: http://nutritionfacts.org/video/treating-parkinsons-disease-with-diet]

Planting helps prevent Parkinson's, with coffee being a star performer. Not only is plants-only vitamin C a strong antioxidant, it's vital as a co-factor in dopamine production, so less Parkinson's for Planters and more well-being.

Exercise boosts dopamine and norepinephrine levels too, almost instantaneously. Perhaps we should all walk to the coffee shop and back every day?

The exercise would benefit obese people who've not only developed insulin resistance, requiring more pancreatic release of insulin, but also resistance to dopamine's effect on the brain pleasure center, requiring more and more fat or sugar for a diminishing return of happiness. Fat and sugar are now known to be addictive, and fat 'n' sugar highs are just like other highs – junkies always need to up the dose.

Anhedonia – the inability to experience pleasure – is part of an eating disorder that is a vicious circle of eating non-foods and becoming fatter and becoming unhappier and eating more to dull the unhappiness. Dietary anhedonia via dopamine resistance can spill over into our sex lives too, already compromised in Meaters by insufficient genital blood supply. Erectile dysfunction and decreased dopamine sensitivity are a powerful recipe for Meater unhappiness.

Planting breaks the dopamine deficiency cycle. Unlike people who practice omnivorism, Planters have no spurious dilemma. Planters eat only food.

Meating and Junking are dopamine-deficiency diseases.

33. Neurotransmitters, part 3: adrenaline (epinephrine)

Please note that my opinion on adrenaline is entirely speculative. I have zero information to back this up.

Webster's College Dictionary describes epinephrine as:

"1. a hormone secreted by the adrenal medulla upon stimulation by the central nervous system in response to stress, as anger or fear, and acting to increase heart rate, blood pressure, cardiac output, and carbohydrate metabolism.

2. a commercial preparation of this substance, used chiefly as a heart stimulant and antiasthmatic.

Also called adrenaline."

Adrenaline is animals' "fight or flight hormone."

Without any proof, and absolutely open to being proven wrong, I'm as certain as I can be that terrified animals in slaughterhouses, all of whom are conscious, after being 'stunned' by a captive bolt gun, while they're being dismembered – a truly awful word – release copious quantities of adrenaline, a goodly portion of which we eat when we're Meaters. I can't imagine that the outcome is beneficial. If dietary adrenaline is responsible for Meater aggression, I wouldn't be surprised.

By the way, using adrenaline from animals (or a facsimile thereof) to treat asthma caused by eating animals is bizarre form of homeopathy – using like to treat like. I guess it doesn't occur to Meaters that to stop Meating is the cure, any more than fish find water problematic.

Strictly speaking, adrenaline doesn't belong in this section of animal deficiencies. I'll admit, yet again, that adrenaline may or may not be a physical health issue. If it is, it's an overload issue, not a deficiency.

The deficiency is a deficiency of heart, a metaphysical ignore-ance of others' needs. Not ignorance. Everyone knows how animals suffer. At this late stage of the Holocaust of the Animals, "But I didn't know…" doesn't cut it any more, if it ever did.

I hope you've finally realized this, René Descartes, wherever you are.

A keen vivisectionist, Descartes thought the howls of the living dogs he carved up the mere reflexes of insensate mechanisms. "Cogito, ergo sum," and they don't cogitate. Has Descartes' "I think, therefore I am" been the most disastrous mantra we humans ever adopted? (Or was it our willful transformation of a benevolent Biblical "Dominion" into our birthright to dominate all others?) Fortunately for our non-human sisters and brothers, saner, kinder dicta are arising: I feel, therefore I am. I love, I play, I grieve, I know fear and joy; therefore I am worthy of consideration and respect.

Meating is an empathy-deficiency disease.

Now let's look at some of the Eatiological mechanisms of Meating …

Planter mechanisms of optimal health in which Meating is deficient

That's it for substances in which Meating and Junking are deficient. I'm sure there are others, but "that'll do, Pig, that'll do," as Farmer Arthur H. Hoggett said to Babe.

In section 2 we learned about many mechanisms by which Meating causes ill-health. Now I'm going to list some nutrition mechanisms of good health which are available when we're Planters but which are unavailable to Meaters.

Think of yin and yang; joined opposites; a dialectic between the positives of Planting and the mirrored negatives of Meating. For example, animals are pro-oxidative. Eating them promotes free radical formation, or oxidation. Plants are antioxidants – they counter the effects of Meating and Junking by dousing free radicals. Animals and Junk are seriously deficient in antioxidants.

Among the following few listings are qualities that plants have and animals don't. In effect, I'm just listing the opposite effects of what Meating causes. Meating causes problems like oxidative stress, ischemia, inflammation, so animals are deficient in their opposites, antioxidants, anti-ischemics and anti-inflammatories.

For whatever Meating causes, Planting has a remedy.

34. Antioxidants

Plants are antioxidants. Put another way, antioxidants are plants. If they occur in animals, they're there because the animals ate them (except for uric acid – an endogenous antioxidant so potent that we need to minimize our levels.) To eat animals to get at the antioxidants they got from eating plants is a perversion of nutrition sense. (Cough, cough… the same can be said of animal proteins.)

35. Anti-inflammatories

By and large, plants which counter oxidation also counter inflammation. Oxidation causes inflammation. When we eat them, animals cause inflammation, either through the direct action of animal proteins on arthritic joints, for example, or via Neu5Gc, "the inflammatory meat molecule," or by disrupting our colon's gut flora. (When the Meater wrecking ball swings into action, there are usually multiple pathways it takes.)

Animals are lovely, but they're not food. I love them, so I don't love eating them. I don't love "my meat" – it's not mine, it's theirs. It's their muscles. Meat is an artificial construct in human nutrition. Meat as food only exists for omnivores and carnivores, which it has been the aim of this entire book to prove that we are not.

36. Anticarcinogens

Anticarcinogens are mostly plants, just like the antioxidants. Just as most antioxidants are also anti-inflammatory, there's also wide overlap with anticarcinogens. One Bing cherry or one cling peach to rule them all.

The merest stub of a Wikipedia entry says: "An anticarcinogen (also known as a **carcinopreventive agent**) is a substance that **counteracts the effects of a carcinogen or inhibits the development of cancer.** Anticarcinogens are different from anticarcinoma agents (also known as anticancer or anti-neoplastic agents) in that anticarcinoma agents are used to selectively destroy or inhibit cancer cells after cancer has developed. Interest in anticarcinogens is motivated primarily by the principle that it is preferable to prevent disease (**preventive medicine**) than to have to treat it (**rescue medicine**).

When consumed as part of a low fat diet, fiber-containing **grain products, fruits, and vegetables** may reduce the risk of some types of cancer."

Exactly. Well said. Preventive medicine via Planting. Eggs, animal flesh, fishes and dairy will never, ever, ever be categorized as anticarcinogens.

And what is a true low-fat diet? It's a no-animal diet.

Whole grains are a great source of phytates, powerful anticarcinogens. As Michael Greger says:

> "Unlike most other anti-cancer agents, the phytates naturally found in whole plant foods may trigger **cancer cell differentiation**, causing them to revert back to behaving more like normal cells."

[See: http://nutritionfacts.org/video/phytates-for-rehabilitating-cancer-cells/]

(Planting, by removing the cause of cancer, can restore normal function in cancerous cells, while starving carcinomas of sugar is to kill them while targeting a cancer symptom, as we saw with Dr. Joseph Mercola earlier.)

Another antioxidant anticarcinogen is the curcumin in cooked turmeric, which boosts the activity of an enzyme called catalase, which can destroy millions of oxidative molecules per second. High turmeric consumption in curries is probably why Indian cancer rates have historically been so low. Low animal consumption doesn't hurt.

As well as being carcinogenic, Meating is an anticarcinogen-deficiency disease. So is Junking.

37. Anti-angiogenesis agents

Continuing with cancer… There are phytonutrients such as **apigenin, fisitin** and **luteolin** that prevent tumors from growing blood vessels to supply themselves with nutrients. These phytonutrients starve cancers, prevent them from growing, and kill them.

Fisitin may be why strawberries are protective against esophageal cancer; the other two are found in most plants, particularly citrus fruits and peppers.

Meating promotes inflammation; inflammation promotes angiogenesis. PhIP, Kathy Freston's "three strikes breast carcinogen" is particularly involved in Meating's carcinogenesis.

Meating is both an angiogenic and an anti-angiogenic-deficiency disease.

38. Aromatase inhibitors

Most breast cancer cells thrive on estrogen. Many of them are able to make their own estrogen out of testosterone, via aromatase, an enzyme. Mushrooms act as aromatase inhibitors, blocking estrogen formation, blocking breast tumor growth.

Animals supply the hormones that cause the cancer; plants (fungi, in this case) inhibit the hormones.

Meating is an aromatase inhibitor deficiency disease.

39. DNA repair enzymes

Continuing the Planter anti-cancer theme (or the Meater cancer theme)… Earlier we saw that amazing, plants-only chlorophyll is a "carcinogen interceptor," blocking mutagens from mutating our DNA and causing cancer. And plant antioxidant fire jumpers prevent DNA damage too by putting out free radical forest fires.

But what happens if carcinogenesis does begin? Can we repair our DNA?

Yes. There are phytonutrients that upregulate our genes to create more DNA repair enzymes – epigenetics in action, beneficially promoted by

Planting, via a home-made protein called P53 which binds to our DNA and mobilizes the DNA repair enzymes.

Planting (especially of berries) is what gets our repair enzymes cracking. Meating is a DNA repair enzyme deficiency disease.

40. Epigenetic up- and down-regulators

Populations of people who've long lived in association with grains have more copies of genes for digesting grains. They've evolved over eons to be efficient "starchivores." These are genetic adaptations.

Epigenetic changes are changes in gene expression without changing the physical genes themselves. We arrive in this world with our genes in place, but it's up to us whether we switch them on or leave them off. Genes get switched on and off through environmental interactions, and by now we should know that our most powerful environmental interactions occur thrice daily (if we're privileged Westerners) at breakfast, lunch and supper.

Foods and non-foods are the environment, up close and in our faces.

Eating food causes beneficial epigenetic changes all around. Meating and Junking cause epigenetic havoc. For example, after Dr. Dean Ornish proved that Planting can reverse prostate cancer in 2005, he showed in 2008 how Planting flipped the switches of hundreds of genes to new, beneficial settings to reverse cancer.

Ornish D, Magbanua MJ, Weidner G, Weinberg V, Kemp C, Green C, Mattie MD, Marlin R, Simko J, Shinohara K, Haqq CM, Carroll PR. Changes in prostate gene expression in men undergoing an intensive nutrition and lifestyle intervention. *Proc Natl Acad Sci U S A.* 17;105(24):8369-74, 2008.

(*The Proceedings of the National Academy of Sciences* (*PNAS*) is one serious scientific journal – the likes of ex-journalists Gary Taubes, Bryan Walsh and Nina Teicholz don't get published there.)

On the other hand, POPs like pesticides can cause cancer directly through DNA damage or through detrimental epigenetic changes in gene expression. It's as if a drunken singer mangles a song either by changing the words altogether or by slurring them so badly they can't be understood.

Genetics isn't destiny. What we eat is far more important. Planting trumps genes, 9 times out of 10. Genetics is passé; epigenetics rules.

Low-Carb Bullshit Artists hate epigenetics, just like they hate epidemiology, because neither branch of science tells them what they want to hear. In fact, epidemiology shows the exact opposite of what Meaters want to hear: that Planting prevents degenerative "diseases" and obesity, and creates ideal conditions for longevity; and then epigenetics provides one of the mechanisms whereby Planting causes positive outcomes and Meating, negative.

At each meal we can make a choice between eating ourselves epigenetically healthy with Plants. Or we can eat ourselves sick, as Meaters and Junkers.

Meating is an epigenetic sinkhole.

41. IGF-1 Binding Proteins
Still on carcinogenesis…

When we eat animals, animal proteins stimulate our livers to release IGF-1, our growth hormone, and our body is told to build, build, build. This is only supposed to happen in human neonates when our mothers feed us breast milk. Mother's milk proteins are the only animal proteins we're supposed to receive during our entire lifetimes. Okay, faced with this aberration – animals stampeding through our blood – our livers churn out IGF-1.

Another thing happens too: our levels of IGF-1-BP go down. BP stands for binding proteins, and their role is to remove carcinogenic growth hormones and steroid sex hormones like estrogen and testosterone from circulation. But, faced with animal amino acid building blocks to get rid of, the levels of IGF-1- BP plummet, further worsening IGF-1's carcinogenic effect.

Planters naturally have the healthy reverse condition: low IGF-1 levels and high liver and blood levels of IGF-1- BP. The higher our binding protein levels are, the more we're protected against cancer.

Meating is an IGF-binding protein deficiency disease.

42. Brown fat and the thermogenic effect
Meaters lack 'plant calories.' Of course, there's no such thing. What happens is this: Planting raises our metabolic rate slightly, shifting more calories to be burned as heat rather than stored as fat. This is known as the thermogenic effect, and it accounts for roughly a difference of 0.4 – 0.5kg (~1 pound) in body weight per year between Planters and Meaters on an isocaloric (equal energy) diet.

Meaters create more abdominal white fat, implicated in meatabolic syndrome. Planters create more brown fat, which is sparsely laid down over the neck and shoulder area, and which is burned to create heat.

Meating is a brown fat deficiency disease; a thermogenic inefficiency disease.

43. Adiponectin

Continuing with obesity… Adiponectin is a hormone which is protective against "gynoid lipodystrophy," aka cellulite. High adiponectin levels = low butt fat. (High butter fat = high butt fat.)

Meating drops our adiponectin levels by almost 20%. Planting raises them by almost 20%.

Meating is an adiponectin-deficiency disease.

Cellulite isn't a feminist issue; it's a Meater issue.

44. Leptin and ghrelin

According to Wikipedia: "Leptin (from Greek λεπτός leptos, "thin"), the "satiety hormone," is a hormone made by adipose cells that helps to regulate energy balance by inhibiting hunger. Leptin is opposed by the actions of the hormone ghrelin, the "hunger hormone." Both hormones… regulate appetite... In obesity, a decreased sensitivity to leptin occurs, resulting in an inability to detect satiety despite high energy stores." When we're overweight, our bodies can't tell we're full even when we're stuffed.

I find it fascinating that it's the fat cells themselves that release these two hormones that tell us whether *they're* hungry or not! Talk about minds of their own.

So, these two hormone antagonists duke it out constantly, satiety (fullness) vs. hunger. When we're obese, our bodies become resistant to leptin, the satiety hormone, (in much the same way that we become resistant to another hormone, insulin), and ghrelin – Mr. Hunger – wins, so we eat more and we gain weight.

What boosts leptin levels? Planting. What drops leptin levels? Meating. Planting leads to skinny people; Meating leads to fat. Leptin/ghrelin is one of the Eatiology mechanisms that explains the epidemiology of skinny Planters and overweight Meaters.

Meating is a leptin deficiency disease.

45. Mineral absorption enhancers & 'dis-enhancers'

We've seen that several minerals are absorbed differently depending on whether they come packaged in animals or plants. Animal iron and animal phosphorus are notable rebels, refusing to obey limits. Plant mineral absorption, on the other hand, is much easier for our bodies to regulate, sometimes with better absorption (e.g. calcium); some plant nutrients like phytates may slightly decrease iron and zinc absorption, while vitamin C boosts iron absorption from plants. Meating lacks this finesse – Meater iron blows through our gut walls regardless of whether we have enough or not.

There are phytonutrients that behave as mineral absorption enhancers – the entire allium family, which includes garlic, onions, leeks, scallions, spring onions and shallots.

Unregulated heme iron absorption causes oxidative stress; phosphorus overload can lead to kidney damage; and systemic acidosis leads to muscle wasting as calcium is stripped from our muscles (not our bones) to buffer acid. There are no Meater mechanisms which advance or retard mineral absorption the way that the onion family, phytates and vitamin C do.

Meating is a mineral absorption regulator deficiency disease.

46. Detoxification enzymes

There's something about broccoli and it's cruciferous cousins, cabbage, kale, Brussels sprouts and others, that upregulates our livers' production of detoxification enzymes. It's probably the cancer-busting sulforaphane. Berries do the same thing, causing our livers to clean house (that is, more than they already do, all the time.)

Animals supply the toxins; plants supply the detox enzymes.

47. Xenohormesis

When plants are stressed they produce antioxidants and anti-inflammatories. This process of producing beneficial substances to cope with bad situations is known as hormesis. We take advantage of plant hormesis by eating the plants and getting *their* anti-stress phytonutrients. We're the xeno- foreigners practicing xenohormesis.

When animals are stressed they produce adrenaline and stress hormones and, probably, metabolites of metaphysical compounds known as "anguish" when their calves are stolen from them and "bewilderment and terror" as they go to slaughter.

Meating is a xenohormesis (and compassion) deficiency disease.

48. Apoptosis

Apoptosis is "programmed cell death." Our immune systems clear cancer cells from our systems, alerting them when it's time to die. On a constant diet of animals, cancer cells become immortal, dividing and metastasizing. Planting boosts apoptosis.

Meating is an apoptosis-deficiency condition.

49. Natural killer cells

Berries are outstanding at increasing the numbers of our immune system's natural killer cells, vital for defense against cancer. Other immune components need to meet up with an antigen before our bodies start manufacturing clones of the antibodies needed to combat the intruder. NK cells are our standing army; the rest are reserves and new recruits, enlisted on demand.

We have billions of NK cells constantly circulating through us, on the lookout for intruders. Some phytonutrients in berries (and the spice cardamom) can double the number of NK cells we have, thus boosting our immunity.

Planting confers high levels of immune function. Meating confers an immunocompromised condition.

50a. Small intestine immune system activators: Aryl receptors

This book is about why animals aren't food, and, if there are 50 Ways to Leave Your Lover, then there are 50 Ways to Retrieve Your Liver in this Animal Deficiency section.

> "Just snip out the back bacon, Jack
> Make an eggless diet plan, Stan
> You don't eat the koi, Roy
> Just set the chickens free
> Stay off the pus, Gus
> You won't feel disgust much
> Just drop off the turkey, Lee
> And get yourself free."

With apologies to Paul Simon.

Pigs, chicken's eggs, fishes, cow's milk, turkeys… none of them is food.

For the last two entries in this Meater deficiency section, I'd like us to put on our evolutionary biologist hats (or our creationist hats, if we'd prefer). It doesn't matter which.

We've established that the time the environment impinges on us the most is when things we've eaten are a single enterocyte cell's width away from our real innards. To facilitate absorption of nutrients, these gut cells must let the environment in, and wastes out, all the time.

Eating is when we're at maximum danger of environmental poisoning, so it's natural that our immune systems should be at DefCon1 while we're eating. Right? We need our immune system to be on high alert, looking out for would-be assassins and saboteurs. Between meals our immuneteers can relax and stand down.

What activates our small intestine immune system when we eat? That should be obvious. Animals. They're the most endotoxin-, pollutant-, parasite- and pathogen-encrusted things we eat. Our bodies have to know straight away when crut-filled animals hit town.

Except... plants are our immune system activators, not animals.

Now, while some Meaters might crow, saying: See, plants are so bad for us, they cause our immune systems to be flashing red, that's not right. As I've shown over and over, whole plants bring nothing but benefits, unless contaminated by animals.

We're either the culmination of billions of years of incremental evolution or God's sudden creation. Either way, activation of our intestinal tract's immune system only by plants shows that we are adapted to eating plants only. Would either God or evolution have enabled us to eat animals without activating our gut's immune systems? Does that make any sense?

Animals are far and away the dirtiest things we put in our mouths. Or do Meaters think early hominins always ate an hors d'oeuvre of grass to activate gut immunity before chowing down on a stegosaurus steak?

We know that Planters have superior immune function and that Meaters have compromised immune function, by comparison. And Planting primes the small intestine's immune pump.

This is how it works:

Intraepithelial lymphocytes (IELs) are small, round white blood cells, immune system components that live between the epithelial cells that make up the mucosal lining of our gastrointestinal (GI) tracts. (Our reproductive tracts too.) Their surfaces are covered with receptors known as aryl hydrocarbon (Ah) receptors. They're the ignition switch for starting up our immune system motors, and the key is plants, particularly cruciferous vegetables such as broccoli, cabbage, cauliflower and kale.

What this means, in evolutionary biology terms, is that we humans (and the species before us) grew up over millions of years in tight association with the plant kingdom, with not enough animal input to change our basic frugivore, herbivore, starchivore, plantivore, phytophage genetic makeup. We lack the genetic code, even now, after geological ages of eating animals, for Meating to activate our intraepithelial response the way that Planting does. Our ancestors ate plants for so long before we started to eat animals that we'd already established how to alert our immune system to incoming food… with plants.

We saw confirmatory evidence with chlorophyll, how our blood and plant blood are almost identical; heme and chlorophyll. Further evidence of our non-Meater nature is that atherosclerosis is an immune response to Meating. If anyone can name me one omnivore or carnivore that forms atherosclerotic plaques in response to animal cholesterol, I'll give them a small house. There aren't any. The notion of human nutritional exceptionalism is a costly one, with millions of us ignorantly succumbing to Meating each year.

The overwhelming tower of evidence for our Planter nature, listed throughout the pages of this book, is capped by this semi-final piece of the puzzle; plants activate our small intestine's immune function when we eat them; not animals. Plants and humans go together like two peas in a pod.

It's clear that we're Planters.

Meating is an immune system activator deficiency disease.

50b. Immune system deactivators in the colon: T_{regs}

In Part 1B (Mechanisms), under Deranged gut flora, I described how beneficial bacteria colonize our colons when we feed them on a high-fiber, whole-plant diet. We feed our bacterial digestive-and-immune 'organ' on fiber and phytates and other phytonutrients, and in return they make nutrients for us and they regulate the colon's immune function and prevent cancer.

One Meater deficiency may lead to another. Continuing with the thread I started earlier in this Animal MIAs section, discussing Planter deficiencies in fiber, phytates, gut flora, propionate, lignans and butyrate, out greatest Meater deficiency may come as a result of suppressing *Faecalibacterium prausnitzii*, and other beneficial colon bacteria like the 'clostridial clusters' who've been living as part of the human intestines for millions of years.

One of the many reasons why Meaters have worse immune function (and more inflammation) in the colon – and are thus more susceptible to inflammatory bowel and leaky gut conditions such as ulcerative colitis, Crohn's "disease" and colorectal cancer – is because Meaters create conditions which are inhospitable to our fiber-eating bacteria.

The final deficiency in my list of 50 comes at the end of this chain:

Low fiber diets (Meating and Junking) $\rightarrow$ $\downarrow$ *F. prausnitzii* et al $\rightarrow$ $\downarrow$ butyrate and other fatty-acid production $\rightarrow$ $\downarrow$ Regulatory T cell, or T_{reg} production.

Meating and Junking combine to cause a T_{reg} deficiency disease.

Aryl receptors in our small intestine *activate* our immune system when they perceive a threat. In our colons, T_{regs} actively *suppress* our immune system. They keep the immune system from attacking our intestinal flora.

Remember, our intestinal flora are us. They're a vital part of us, tantamount to a bodily organ. Therefore, when we eat low-fiber (low-whole-carb, high-animal) diets we're causing an auto-immune response in our colons. We make our immune systems attack other parts of ourselves; in this case, our intestinal bacteria. Animals and junk aren't food… not for us, and not for our bacterial fellow travelers.

Meating is a form of unintentional slow-motion self-murder, as opposed to suicide, which stems from a conscious desire to do away with one's self. If somnambulists are sleepwalkers, Meaters and Junkers are "somnophages" – sleep-eaters. We don't know how to eat. We eat ourselves to death, in part because we eat our multi-part bacterial gut organs to death. And we're oblivious to the fact that we're doing it.

Animals and junked plants aren't food.

Sidebar: On PREbiotics, PRObiotics and 'RETRObiotics'

Vegetarians and other non-vegans make much of the probiotics they get from eating the refrigerated, fruit-flavored goop otherwise known as yogurt.

WebMD says "Probiotics are live bacteria and yeasts that are good for your health, especially your digestive system. We usually think of bacteria as something that causes diseases. But your body is full of bacteria, both good and bad. Probiotics are often called "good" or "helpful" bacteria because they help keep your gut healthy."

Probiotics are supplements that Meaters and Junkers have to take to artificially create a healthy microbiome, because their diets are devoid of the fiber upon which a healthy gut bacteria population thrives.

Yogurt is bacterially fermented milk. Being fermented, it's got less lactose in it, so it's not as terrible for us as regular milk. But it's still milk. It's just as laden with animal hormones, animal fats and animal proteins, and just as contaminated with environmental pollutants. It's not food for humans, or for cows. No cow has ever wittingly fed a fermented milk culture to her calf, and no adult cow drinks any kind of milk.

Probiotics are, in effect, retrobiotics. We add them to our diet to retrofit our bacteria, while we wipe out the same bacteria with other parts of our diet: animals and junk.

(It's like Low-Carb Bullshit Artists with diabetes having to take metformin to control their Meater-induced diabetes.) If we quit Meating and Junking, we can quit taking probiotics (and metformin and statins and… and… and…)

Prebiotics, on the other hand, are just whole plants, packed full of fiber and fiber-associated nutrients. They're food for humans and food for bacteria. They feed us all. Prebiotics aren't supplements; they're merely whole food.

That said, Meaters and Junkers would be well-advised to carry on swallowing their probiotics and their drugs to make up for the ill-effects of their immune- and otherwise deficient diets.

Those of us who'd prefer to live long healthy lives should ditch the yogurt, and just eat the fruit.

Stop Press Bonus Meater Deficiencies

51. Natural Products That Target Cancer Stem Cells

Here's an exciting paper, out in November 2015, just in time to make it into the first edition of this book early in 2016:

Moselhy J, Srinivasan S, Ankem MK, Damodaran C. Natural Products That Target Cancer Stem Cells. *Anticancer Res.* 2015 Nov;35(11):5773-88.

"The cancer stem cell model suggests that tumor initiation is governed by a small subset of distinct cells with stem-like character termed cancer stem cells (CSCs). CSCs possess properties of self-renewal and intrinsic survival mechanisms that contribute to resistance of tumors to most chemotherapeutic drugs. The failure to eradicate CSCs during the course of therapy is postulated to be the driving force for tumor recurrence and metastasis."

Cancer stem cells are resistant to chemotherapy. Not only does chemo not kill CSCs – it can make them more virulent.

This is really important: "Recent studies evaluating NPs against CSC support the **epidemiological evidence linking plant-based diets with reduced malignancy rates**."

Epidemiology shows Planters get less cancer. Here's just one of the many reasons why... **Planters get less cancer because Planting wipes out Cancer Stem Cells.**

Moselhy et al list 25 Natural Products (NPs) that selectively target cancer stem cells, without harming normal cells:

1. Baicalein – Chinese skullcap [Chinese herb of the mint family]
2. β-Carotene – Carrots, leafy greens
3. Curcumin – Turmeric
4. Cyclopamine – Corn lily [not to be eaten – a lethal teratogen]
5. Delphinidin – Blueberry, raspberry
6. Epigallocatechin-3-gallate (EGCG) – Green tea
7. Flavonoids (Genistein) – Soy, red clover, coffee
8. 6-Gingerol – Ginger
9. Gossypol – Cottonseed [not to be eaten – may cause paralysis; sometimes used in China as a male contraceptive]
10. Guggulsterone – Commiphora (myrrh tree)
11. Isothiocyanates – Cruciferous vegetables
12. Linalool – Mint
13. Lycopene – Grapefruit, tomato
14. Parthenolide – Feverfew
15. Perylill alcohol – Mint, cherry, lavender
16. Piperine – Black pepper
17. Placycodon saponin – Playycodon grandifloruim [Chinese bellflower]
18. Psoralidin [a coumarin] – Psoralea corylilyfolia [Babchi, in Ayurveda]
19. Quercetin – Capers, onions
20. Resveratrol – Grapes, plums, berries [not red wine – carcinogenic]
21. Salinomycin – Streptomyces albus [a bacterium which generates mycelia]
22. Silibinin – Milk thistle
23. Ursolic acid – Thyme, basil, oregano
24. Vitamin D3 – [Sunlight on skin] Fish, egg yolk, beef, cod liver oil
25. Withaferin A – Withania somnifera (ashwagandha) [Indian ginseng, a nightshade, also used in Ayurveda.]

What do we notice about all these anti-cancer stem cell agents? With the exception of #24, which is best obtained by the action of sunlight on human skin, they're all plants; not necessarily edible plants, but plants all the same. All the animal products suggested in #24 as sources of vitamin D3 are themselves carcinogenic, so we'd be better off getting D3 from fortified non-junk-foods or a supplement, in the case of us not getting enough sunshine. We should stock up with this vital hormone whenever we can – on holiday, or during non-wintry months.

The reason why chemotherapy is a poor treatment of cancer, and why regression is so common after traditional therapies, is that they tend to kill the cancer daughter cells and so reduce tumor size, but they leave the stem cells untouched, leading to the false hope that the tumor is going, as it shrinks, while the cancer 'seeds' are left to germinate again later.

Using these Natural Products goes right to the root of the cancer, wiping out the stem cells. Plus… they boost our immune systems, which conventional "treatments" such as chemo and radiation are notorious for eradicating. We know that whole plants and their phytonutrients can synergize powerfully. Knowing this, we should eat a wide variety of plants that contain these (and other yet-to-be-discovered) NP substances such as gingerols, isothiocyanates, flavonoids and carotenes, all washed down with a nice cup of EGCG, for spectacularly, synergistically beneficial results. I'd pick them over chemo or radiation every time. [I'm not giving medical advice; merely pointing out the power of the new medicine: lifestyle medicine. Please consult a physician, preferably one versed in nutrition.]

Because we're sweet solar-powered beings (via sunlight and plants), Meating is a sunlight-deficiency condition, lacking in the natural, healing plant products that combat cancer stem cells.

Meating is not only carcinogenic; it's a Natural Product-deficiency disease.

52. Primordial prevention

If "The purpose of primary prevention is to limit the incidence of disease by controlling causes and risk factors," as says Sorin Ursoniu, MD, PhD, then primordial prevention begins even earlier: "Primordial prevention deals with underlying conditions leading to exposure to causative factors."

Planting is automatically primordially preventative of degenerative "diseases".

Why? Because Meating and Junking *are the risk factors* for most chronic ailments.

Meating and Junking are primordial prevention disaster zones.

Summary of MIAs

To aid my summary of missing-in-action animal nutrients [oxymoron alert] and MIA beneficial health mechanisms, I'm going to refer to a 2014 paper by Jennifer Di Noia PhD:

Defining Powerhouse Fruits and Vegetables: A Nutrient Density Approach. *Preventing Chronic Disease* 2014:11:130390 [downloadable at http://www.cdc.gov/pcd/issues/2014/pdf/13_0390.pdf],

In her paper, Dr Di Noia writes: "This article describes a classification scheme defining PFV [**powerhouse fruits and vegetables**] on the basis of **17 nutrients of public health importance** per the Food and Agriculture Organization of the United Nations and Institute of Medicine (i.e., potassium, fiber, protein, calcium, iron, thiamin, riboflavin, niacin, folate, zinc, and vitamins A, B_6, B_{12}, C, D, E, and K)" (3).

Her reference (3) is to Drewnonwski A. Concept of a nutritious food: toward a nutrient density score. *Am J Clin Nutr* 2005;82(4):721-32.

Let's take a look at Dr Di Noia's 17 nutrients "of public health importance":

> calcium
> fiber
> iron
> potassium
> protein
> vit. A (retinol, retinal, and 4 carotenoids incl. beta carotene)
> vitamin B_1 (thiamine)
> vit. B_2 (riboflavin)
> vit. B_3 (niacin)
> vit. B_6 (pyridoxine)
> vit. B_9 (folate)
> vit. B_{12} (cyano-, hydroxy- or methylcobalamin)
> vit. C (ascorbic acid)
> vit. D (cholecalciferol (D_3), ergocalciferol (D_2))
> vit. E (tocopherols, tocotrienols)
> vit. K (phylloquinone, menaquinones)
> zinc

Magnesium doesn't make the list. That surprises me. Just upping our magnesium levels with a few nuts and seeds a day could prevent tens of thousands of fatal heart attacks in the US annually. I guess the FAO had to draw the line somewhere. I think they stopped one nutrient too soon.

This list contains two nutrients we should never, ever get from animals: **iron** and **protein**. As I've shown repeatedly, heme iron and animal protein are extremely toxic carcinogens, via nitrosamines and IGF-1 respectively.

To their detriment, there is no **fiber** in processed animals or plants.

Calcium and **potassium** are far better absorbed and regulated from plants than from animals; calcium from leafy greens, potassium from bananas, beans and nuts.

Zinc can be a problem for vegans: animal zinc is more absorbable than plant zinc (not necessarily a good thing). Plus, as we'd expect with metal accumulation increasing up the "food" chain, animals have lots of zinc in them, with oysters at #1. (The loss of zinc in ejaculate is part of what gives oysters their reputation as aphrodisiacs.) Getting at the zinc from oysters without also getting the PCBs, dioxins and heavy metals is problematic. "Food is a package deal." Planters should just eat plenty of grains, beans, nuts and seeds: food. Plant zinc and iron become more bioaccessible when eaten with "mineral absorption enhancers" such as garlic and onions.

Of the vitamins, **B$_9$** (folate), **C** and **E** are found only in plants; **D** is made by the action of sunlight on human and other animal skin.

Vitamin K comes overwhelmingly from leafy green vegetables. The top 100 sources in the National Nutrient Database list for vit. K doesn't contain a single animal item that's not a Chinese restaurant dish that also contains confounding veggies.

The top sources of **vitamin A** are animals, but there's plenty in dark green leafies, and in yellow, orange and red veggies. Deficiency in the 1st World is almost unheard of, so there's no reason to poison ourselves with animals to get it. As with several other animal issues such as protein, the problem with vitamin A is getting too much, rather than too little.

There's also plenty of **vitamin B$_{12}$** in animals, but unfortunately we'd have to eat the animals to get the B$_{12}$, which is the health equivalent of eating monkey droppings to get at an undigested peanut: the peanut's tasty, but not worth eating shit for.

Which leaves four B vitamins, 1, 2, 3 and 6; thiamine, riboflavin, niacin and pyridoxine. (The other two B vitamins, vitamin B5 (pantothenic acid) and vitamin B7 (biotin) are the only two of the 13 acknowledged vitamins not to make it into this exclusive list of "17 nutrients of public health importance," probably because they don't play hard to get.)

This 2011 study, in which 13,292 people took part, compared the diets of vegetarians to non-vegetarians:

(B. Farmer, B. T. Larson, V. L. Fulgoni III, A. J. Rainville, G. U. Liepa. A vegetarian dietary pattern as a nutrient-dense approach to weight management: An analysis of the national health and nutrition examination survey 1999-2004. *J Am Diet Assoc.* 2011 111(6):819 – 827, abstract available at http://www.ncbi.nlm.nih.gov/pubmed/21616194.)

Farmer et al start by saying: "Population-based studies have shown that vegetarians have lower body mass index than non-vegetarians, suggesting that vegetarian diet plans may be an approach for weight management. However, a perception exists that vegetarian diets are deficient in certain nutrients."

In other words, we Meaters think you semi-Planter vegetarians are deficient in a bunch of stuff. Let's see if that's true.

Instead, they found that **"Mean intakes of fiber, vitamins A, C, and E, thiamin, riboflavin, folate, calcium, magnesium, and iron were higher for all vegetarians than for all non-vegetarians."**

Better in every single nutrient tested, including calcium and iron. Also more magnesium: fewer sudden cardiac deaths.

That takes care of **vitamins B$_1$ and B$_2$.** The people who ate the fewest animals had the best thiamin and riboflavin levels. Not optimal, but better – after all these were vegetarians, not vegans.

The researchers concluded: "These findings suggest that vegetarian diets are nutrient dense, consistent with dietary guidelines, and could be recommended for weight management without compromising diet quality."

I think they could have been slightly less underwhelming, considering how much more favorable the results were for mere vegetarians than Meaters.

They could have said, quite truthfully: "A whole-food vegan diet is the most nutrient-dense, and the only logical diet for humans."

624

Next up: niacin.

I'm pleased, as one of part-English descent, to say that the top source of **niacin (B$_3$)** per 100g in the USDA database is "yeast extract spread." That sounds suspiciously like Marmite or Vegemite to me, two yeast extract spreads well known in Britain and the colonies, with the look and acquired taste of coal tar waste, long-fermented in a Scottish peat bog. I eat lots of it, so I'm niacinically sorted. The top database entry per household, a turkey breast weighing 1.1171 kg contains 1.1171 mg of niacin, while 0.984 kg vegetarian stew contains 118.56 mg. The stuff's everywhere in food; we shouldn't have a problem getting enough of it, even if absorption may vary.

Pretty much everyone gets enough **vitamin B$_6$ (pyridoxine),** so I'm not sure why our researchers were more concerned about it than magnesium, of which almost 98% of Americans are deficient. (Hey, wait a minute; almost 2% of the population is now vegan. Is there a connection? Of course, there is. I'm not saying all vegans get enough magnesium, but we're far more likely to when we're vegan.) As with potassium, there's plenty of B$_6$ in bananas, beans and nuts. (Having enough B$_6$, B$_9$ and B$_{12}$ helps keep homocysteine in check, to suppress inflammation, particularly in the brain.)

Summary of the 17 nutrients of concern

If we're rooting for the Meater nutrient team, it's fourth down with 99 yards to go, with seconds on the clock, our 3rd string quarterback just got crocked, so the water boy had to take his place, and our team is trailing by 30 points. It's not a strong position. (Yet people bet on it all the time.)

Just as we saw with the 50 animal deficiencies I noted earlier, getting one's nutrients from animals is either impossible (because they don't contain them) or fraught with danger, if they do: vitamin B$_{12}$ is a good thing; vitamin B$_{12}$ from animals is anything but. Calcium is a necessary thing; calcium from dairy is not.

Of the 17 nutrients studied, only zinc, B$_{12}$ and D may take some thought for Planters to achieve optimal levels. We do this by eating a wide range of whole plants, by taking a daily or weekly B$_{12}$ supplement, and getting enough sun exposure; failing which, a supplement.

For Meaters, problems abound, starting with growth hormone-promoting, carcinogenic animal protein; continuing with free radical-causing, carcinogenic heme iron; going further with fiber-, folate-, C-, E-and K-poor or –absent animals.

In their paper above, published in the staunchly pro-Meater *Journal of the American Dietetic Association*, of all places, Farmer et al showed that the Plantier we are, the better our intake of "fiber, vitamins A, C, and E, thiamin, riboflavin, folate, calcium, magnesium, and iron."

We achieve optimal nutrition when we Plant… with the single exception of the limp noodle with which Meaters try to stove in Planters' heads: vitamin B_{12}.

And yet, eating the whole-food way Planters do, we can remedy all of our nutrition problems simply by taking a harmless tablet once a week while the plants do the rest.

Eating the way Meaters do, we can certainly avoid taking those dreadful B_{12} supplements, sure, but then we'd have to take statins and aspirin and warfarin for our heart conditions, and zoloft or prozac for our depression, and viagra for our erectile dysfunction, and diuretics (water pills) or ACE inhibitors or angiotensin II receptor blockers or beta blockers or calcium channel blockers or renin inhibitors for our hypertension, and metformin for our diabetes (hi, Prof. Noakes), and tamoxifen or aromatase inhibitors for our breast cancer, and fosamax for our osteoporosis, and cetuximab for our metastatic colorectal cancer, and this for our triglycerides, and that for our gout, and the other thing for our kidney stones, and… and… and… all to combat the symptoms of Meating, world without end.

B_{12} is an embarrassing argument to use *in favor of* Meating and *against* Planting.

As we've seen, Meating truly is a nutrient-poor disaster of a diet.

To quote Prof. T. Colin Campbell one more time: "There is no nutrient in animals that's not better supplied by plants…" and there are tens of thousands of plant nutrients of which animals are totally bereft.

If we're humans, we're Planters. Planting is our God- and/or evolution-given nature.

Anyone who needs a little extra convincing should check out Dr. Milton Mills' excellent *The Comparative Anatomy of Eating*. It's available at http://www.adaptt.org/Mills%20The%20Comparative%20Anatomy%20of%20Eating1.pdf

After examining our facial muscles, jaw type, jaw joint location, jaw motion, major jaw muscles, mouth opening vs. head size, teeth (incisors), teeth (canines), teeth (molars), chewing, saliva, stomach type, stomach acidity, stomach capacity, length of small intestine, colon, liver, kidneys and nails (vs. claws), he says:

> "In conclusion, we see that human beings have the gastrointestinal tract structure of a "committed" herbivore. Humankind does not show the mixed structural features one expects and finds in anatomical omnivores such as bears and raccoons. Thus, from comparing the gastrointestinal tract of humans to that of carnivores, herbivores and omnivores we must conclude that humankind's GI tract is designed for a purely plant-food diet."

Planters... that's what we are.

When it comes to the rapid encephalization of *H. & F. sapiens* in our primeval past, my money's on Rachel Carmody and Richard Wrangham, with their theory that the control of fire, which allowed greater energy from cooked plants, particularly the USOs or underground storage organs (such as tubers) which Nathaniel Dominy is so keen on.

Paleonutrition is a stimulating subject. However, it's entirely irrelevant to the study of modern nutrition, for the simple reason that only whole plants are food, to whom and where and when it matters - to us modern human beings, living right here, right now.

Even in the extremely unlikely event that eating animals made us human by causing our sugar-powered brains to put on a growth spurt millennia ago, our digestive tracts and arteries, hearts and brains still can't tolerate animals today. So we should just say thank you to our hominin ancestors whose subsistence on animal emergency rations may have given us our modern brains, and now that we're not constrained in our eating choices, let normal plant-food service resume.

~

Part 5 (Summary): Why Animals Aren't Food

When the Cows Come Home to Roost:
Consequences of Meating

Robert Louis Stevenson: "Everybody, soon or late, sits down to a banquet of consequences."

In Part 1 of this book, ANIMALS, THEMSELVES, I described

- the CONSTITUENTS of animals
- the MECHANISMS whereby Meating sickens us
- the EATIOLOGY of degenerative "diseases", now known to be symptoms of Meating

I showed that Meating and Junking are responsible for 90% of all the "Diseases" of Western Civilization, and that what we think of as diseases are usually reversible symptoms of Meating and Junking.

In Part 2 (~~FOOD~~BORNE PATHOGENS), I described the life forms that come packaged with animals. These include:

- Viruses
- Bacteria and their toxins
- Parasites
- Fungi, including yeasts
- Prions

I showed that Meating is responsible for at least 90% of the illnesses, hospitalizations and deaths due to microbes, because of the extraordinary load of pathogens Meating introduces.

In Part 3 (~~FOOD~~BORNE CONTAMINANTS), I described the inert pollution with which animals become contaminated, including:

- Industrial pollutants, inserted accidentally and
- "Food" and feed additives, contaminants inserted on purpose.

I showed how the biological processes of bio-accumulation and bio-magnification are why Meating introduces more than 90% of environmental pollutants into our bodies.

In Part 4 (ANIMAL DEFICIENCIES), or Missing in Action, I described some of the nutrients that animals and junk lack, including fiber, carbohydrates, vitamins, phytates and other phytonutrients.

I showed that hyper-processed plants and animals have an Eatiology ("disease"-causing effect) that's very similar in many ways. Processed junk behaves more like processed animals than it does like whole plants.

In Part 5 (SUMMARY), it's my intention to put all the pieces together. After one last section of reductionist science - almost seventy pages of references to and discussions of landmark studies in biomedicine - I'm going to switch gears and practice nutrition science as it ought to be practiced - in a holistic or wholistic way.

A Turd's Eye View of an Animal Meal describes what happens when we eat a meal of animals, from when we ingest them to when we excrete them, pointing out the harmful effects they have on our digestion, metabolism and overall health.

After that we'll be well-armed with both reductionist and wholistic nutrition science with which to view the world and to see - because we'll know to the depths of our being that animals aren't food - that as individuals we need to make changes if we'd like to thrive, and that, as a species, we're going to need to make changes if we're to survive.

Here now is the last of the reductionist science...

References: Landmarks in medical and nutrition research

Blaise Pascal is supposed to have apologized to a friend that he hadn't had the time to write a shorter letter. I apologize that five years hasn't been enough time for me to condense everything I wanted to say about Meater and Junker mal-nutrition into fewer than the 800-odd pages it's taken me.

As a result, and because my sources are liberally sprinkled throughout the text, I'm not going to do what Michael Greger did in his *How Not to Die* and supply you with more than a hundred pages of references. In 70-odd pages, I'm going to hit the high notes, and I'm going to provide some commentary too. This section contains references to papers about the biggies like diabetes, hypertension, auto-immune conditions, cancer, stroke, heart "disease" and Alzheimer's but not to studies about more obscure maladies such as ankylosing spondylitis or abdominal aortic aneurysm.

But don't worry: everything's connected… ankylosing spondylitis is an auto-immune condition and, with a few exceptions such as celiac disease and rheumatic heart disease, they're usually ailments with the same Meater Eatiology. And AAA is inseparable from atherosclerosis and hypertension, which are also the same thing – it's not possible to give ourselves one without the other – and we give them to ourselves by Meating and Junking.

What's the most important illness in the world? It's the one we have.

If you'd like to read good primary sources about a condition of interest and I haven't cited it in this reference section or in the body of the book, you could do worse than start where I did five years ago, at nutritionfacts.org. Type in, say, polyps, then follow the links to the videos or articles about your topic; then click on the 'sources' link and read the original papers in *The New England Journal of Medicine* or *The Lancet* or wherever they may lurk.

Now let's take a look at the extraordinary source materials behind the lifestyle medicine and plants-only nutrition renaissance. If you watch carefully, you'll notice that all the best new evidence shows the same thing in two different ways: Meating and Junking make us ill, while Planting prevents, stops or heals what Meating and Junking and other things cause. And please note that we're going to measure real health outcomes here, like reversal of illness and extension of life. We're not merely going to manipulate biomarkers as low-carbers are wont to do.

References to papers on animal and junk components
(with a few pathogens thrown in for good measure)

First, a quick word about scientific language. Scientists, like judges, hate to have their opinions overturned on appeal, so they speak circumspectly. We shouldn't be fooled by their heavy use of words like 'may' and 'can.' In our minds we should substitute 'will' and 'do.'

For example, when G. Brewer says: "This copper is potentially toxic because it may penetrate the blood/brain barrier," we can be darn certain that copper *is* toxic because it *does* enter the brain. And when Abrahamsson et al say: "Diet modifications may be one breast cancer prevention strategy," we know that diet modification (Planting) *is* the best strategy.

I won't pussyfoot around: if the best science tells us it's so, I'll say so. If later, better evidence shows that I'm wrong a time or two, I'll let you know. The overall ill-effects of Meating and Junking will endure the picayune.

Acrylamide
M Stott-Miller, ML Neuhouser, JL Stanford. Consumption of deep-fried foods and risk of prostate cancer. *Prostate.* 2013 73(9):960 – 969.

Stott-Miller et al say that "Regular consumption of select deep-fried foods is associated with increased PCa (prostate cancer) risk."

As a prostate owner, I say acrylamide's a good reason to avoid crispy carbs.

Alpha-gal
SP Commins, TAE Platts-Mills. Delayed anaphylaxis to red meat in patients with IgE specific for galactose alpha-1,3-galactose (alpha-gal). *Curr Allergy Asthma Rep.* 2013 13(1):72 – 77.

"Anaphylaxis is a severe allergic reaction that can be rapidly progressing and fatal... delayed onset anaphylaxis 3-6 hours after ingestion of mammalian food products (e.g., beef and pork)."

For 99% of us, food doesn't do this. The exceptions are a tiny fraction of the population that has an issue with gluten and those with allergies to whole plants such as some nuts or seeds or members of the nightshade family).

Ammonia
A Birkett, J Muir, J Phillips, G Jones, K O'Dea. Resistant starch lowers fecal concentrations of ammonia and phenols in humans. *Am J Clin Nutr.* 1996 May;63(5):766-72.

"...RS [resistant starch] significantly attenuates the accumulation of potentially harmful byproducts of protein fermentation in the human colon."

Resistant starch is found in whole plants and it combats the bacterial formation of ammonia from animal proteins in our intestines.

Amyloid, cholesterol and Alzheimer's

Ortiz D, Shea TB. Apple juice prevents oxidative stress induced by amyloid-beta in culture. *J Alzheimers Dis.* 2004 Feb;6(1):27-30.

"Increased oxidative stress contributes to the decline in cognitive performance during normal aging and in neurodegenerative conditions such as Alzheimer's disease... the antioxidant potential of apple products can prevent Amyloid-beta-induced oxidative damage."

An apple a day... plus berries plus citrus plus... no animals or junk.

B Reed et al. Associations between serum cholesterol levels and cerebral amyloidosis. *JAMA Neurol.* 2014 Feb;71(2):195-200.

"Elevated cerebral Aβ [amyloid-beta] level was associated with cholesterol fractions in a pattern analogous to that found in coronary artery disease."

The same cholesterol that causes heart "disease" helps cause Alzheimer's "disease".

"Animal calories" ~ Brown fat or brown adipose tissue

M Saito, T Yoneshiro. Capsinoids and related food ingredients activating brown fat thermogenesis and reducing body fat in humans. *Curr Opin Lipidol.* 2013 Feb;24(1):71-7.

"As human BAT [brown adipose tissue] may be inducible, a prolonged ingestion of capsinoids would recruit active BAT and thereby increase energy expenditure and decrease body fat. In addition to capsinoids, there are numerous food ingredients that are expected to activate BAT and so be useful for the prevention of obesity in daily life." And they're all in plants. Capsaicin is the hot stuff in chilies.

Animal carbohydrates (lactose and galactose)

A. Stang et al. Adolescent milk fat and galactose consumption and testicular germ cell cancer. *Cancer Epidemiol. Biomarkers Prev.*, 15(11):2189-2195, 2006.

"Recent case-control studies suggested that dairy product consumption is an important risk factor for testicular cancer... Our results suggest that milk fat and/or galactose may explain the association between milk and dairy product consumption and seminomatous testicular cancer."

Got milk? Got ball cancer.

Animal fats (Saturated fats and trans fats)

D Estadella et al. Lipotoxicity: effects of dietary saturated and transfatty acids. *Mediators Inflamm.* 2013;2013:137579.

"The ingestion of excessive amounts of saturated fatty acids (SFAs) and transfatty acids (TFAs) is considered to be a risk factor for cardiovascular diseases, insulin resistance, dyslipidemia, and obesity... The saturated and transfatty acids favor a proinflammatory state leading to insulin resistance. These fatty acids can be involved in several inflammatory pathways, contributing to disease progression in chronic inflammation, autoimmunity, allergy, cancer, atherosclerosis, hypertension, and heart hypertrophy as well as other metabolic and degenerative diseases."

Animals and junk aren't food.

Animal proteins

MF McCarty. Vegan proteins may reduce risk of cancer, obesity, and cardiovascular disease by promoting increased glucagon activity. *Med Hypotheses.* 1999 Dec;53(6):459-85.

"An unnecessarily high intake of essential amino acids – either in the absolute sense or relative to total dietary protein – may prove to be as grave a risk factor for 'Western' degenerative diseases as is excessive fat intake."

The right question to ask about protein isn't "Where do we get it?"

It's "How do we not get too much of it?" or "How do we avoid animal proteins?" Plant proteins are superior.

Arachidonic acid

G Esposito et al. Imaging neuroinflammation in Alzheimer's disease with radiolabeled arachidonic acid and PET. *J Nucl Med.* 2008 Sep;49(9):1414-21.

"Incorporation coefficients (K*) of arachidonic acid (AA) in the brain are increased in a rat model of neuroinflammation, as are other markers of AA metabolism. Data also indicate that neuroinflammation contributes to Alzheimer's disease (AD).... K* for AA is widely elevated in the AD brain…"

AA could stand for "animals alone" instead of arachidonic acid.

Biogenic amines

A. J. Vargas et al. Dietary polyamine intake and risk of colorectal adenomatous polyps. *Am. J. Clin. Nutr.* 2012 96(1):133–141.

"Putrescine, spermidine, and spermine are the polyamines required for human cell growth… This study showed a role for dietary polyamines in colorectal adenoma risk."

Carcinogenic polyamines, or biogenic amines form in the dead flesh we eat.

Bones

Peonim V, Udnoon J. Left subclavian arterioesophageal fistula induced by chicken bone with upper gastrointestinal hemorrhage and unexpected death: report of a case. *J Med Assoc Thai.* 2010 Nov;93(11):1332-5.

"Postmortem examination revealed a chicken bone embedded in middle part of esophagus with fistula between the esophagus and the left subclavian artery."

The fibrous skeleton of plants doesn't kill us.

Calcium

Heaney RP, Weaver CM. Calcium absorption from kale. *Am J Clin Nutr.* 1990 Apr;51(4):656-7.

"Absorption of calcium from intrinsically labeled kale was measured in 11 normal women and compared in these same subjects with absorption of calcium from labeled milk. The average test load was 300 mg. Fractional calcium absorption from kale averaged 0.409… and from milk, 0.321... In contrast with the poor absorption previously reported for spinach calcium, kale, a low-oxalate vegetable, exhibits excellent absorbability for its calcium."

Calcium is better absorbed from low-oxalate plants, plus there's no pus, shit, estrogens, cholesterol, lactose, galactose, saturated butterfat, casein, casomorphins, bacteria, antibiotics or pesticides in organic kale.

Carnitine

RA Koeth et al. Intestinal microbiota metabolism of l-carnitine, a nutrient in red meat, promotes atherosclerosis. *Nat Med.* 2013 Apr 7.

"Intestinal microbiota metabolism of choline/phosphatidylcholine produces trimethylamine (TMA), which is further metabolized to a proatherogenic species, trimethylamine-N-oxide (TMAO). Herein we demonstrate that intestinal microbiota metabolism of dietary L-carnitine, a trimethylamine abundant in red meat, also produces TMAO and accelerates atherosclerosis… Intestinal microbiota may thus participate in the well-established link between increased red meat consumption and CVD risk."

Note: There isn't just a postulated link between Meating and cardiovascular "disease" – there's a "well-established link." Everyone in nutrition seems to understand this except the Low-Carb Bullshit Artists, who'd like us to carry on eating the choline in eggs, poultry, dairy and fishes, and the carnitine in red flesh.

Casein

Karina Arnberg et al. Skim Milk, Whey, and Casein Increase Body Weight and Whey and Casein Increase the Plasma C-Peptide Concentration in Overweight Adolescents.

"Outcomes were BMI-for-age Z-scores (BAZs), waist circumference, plasma insulin, homeostatic model assessment, and plasma C-peptide… high intakes of skim milk, whey, and casein increase BAZs in overweight adolescents and that whey and casein increase insulin secretion."

Milk is food for baby cows, not baby humans. Not adult humans either.

Casomorphin

Z Sun et al. Relation of beta-casomorphin to apnea in sudden infant death syndrome. *Peptides*. 2003 Jun;24(6):937-43.

"Beta-CM is an exogenous bioactive peptide derived from casein, a major protein in milk and milk products, which has opioid activity. Mechanistically, circulation of this peptide into the infant's immature central nervous system might inhibit the respiratory center in the brainstem leading to apnea and death."

Cows' milk causes crib death, a.k.a. SIDS (sudden infant death syndrome). Cows' milk kills human babies.

Ceramide

AB Awad, SL Barta, CS Fink, PG Bradford. Beta-Sitosterol enhances tamoxifen effectiveness on breast cancer cells by affecting ceramide metabolism. *Mol Nutr Food Res.* 2008 52(4):419–426.

"The objective of this study was to investigate the effects of the dietary phytosterol beta-sitosterol (SIT) and the antiestrogen drug tamoxifen (TAM) on cell growth and ceramide (CER) metabolism in… human breast cancer cells."

Drugs and phytonutrients both combat ceramide, a metabolite of saturated fats found in animals and junk.

Cholesterol

Low-Carb Bullshit Artists love to bang on about how cholesterol doesn't cause heart "disease". Okay then, let's take a look instead at cholesterol's role in causing cancer, followed by some examples of phytonutrients that help prevent cancer.

C Danilo, PG Frank. Cholesterol and breast cancer development. *Current Opinion in Pharmacology*. 2012 12(6):677–682.

"Breast cancer is the most commonly occurring type of cancer in the world… laboratory studies… indicate that cholesterol is capable of regulating proliferation, migration, and signaling pathways in breast cancer… The recognition of cholesterol as a factor contributing to breast cancer development identifies cholesterol and its metabolism as novel targets for cancer therapy." Or novel targets for Planting.

BJ Grattan Jr. Plant sterols as anticancer nutrients: Evidence for their role in breast cancer. *Nutrients*. 2013 5(2):359 – 387.

"… specific food components have been identified which are uniquely beneficial in mitigating the risk of specific cancer subtypes. Plant sterols are well known for their effects on blood cholesterol levels… the cholesterol modulating actions of plant sterols may overlap with their anti-cancer actions."

What Meating breaks, Planting fixes.

AS Vadodkar, S Suman, R Lakshmanaswamy, C Damodaran. Chemoprevention of breast cancer by dietary compounds. *Anticancer Agents Med Chem*. 2012 12(10):1185 – 1202.

"… daily consumption of dietary phytochemicals reduces the risk of several cancers."

There are zero studies showing that eating animals helps prevent cancer. Natural Products – "novel potent molecules as anticancer agents" – are found only in plants (24 of which we met on page 620). Are the Low-Carb Bullshit Artists the ultimate misogynists, that they simply refuse to present this information that could save millions of women's lives each year?

Copper

G. J. Brewer. The risks of copper toxicity contributing to cognitive decline in the aging population and to Alzheimer's disease. *Journal of the American College of Nutrition*, 28(3):238, 2009.

"In this brief review I advance the hypothesis that copper toxicity is the major cause of the epidemic of mild cognitive impairment and Alzheimer's disease engulfing our aging population… The epidemic is associated with the use of copper plumbing, and the taking of copper in multi-mineral supplements. Food copper (organic copper) is processed by the liver and is transported and sequestered in a safe manner. Inorganic copper, such as that in drinking water and copper supplements, largely bypasses the liver and enters the free copper pool of the blood directly. This copper is potentially toxic because it may penetrate the blood/brain barrier."

The animals we eat are also often contaminated with inorganic copper from pesticides, particularly in the USA, which is lax about testing for pesticide residues. (Why? Because the USDA and FDA et al cater to corporate interests, not the well-being of the public they're supposed to serve.)

Creatine

Benton D, Donohoe R. The influence of creatine supplementation on the cognitive functioning of vegetarians and omnivores. *Br J Nutr.* 2011 Apr;105(7):1100-5.

"…in vegetarians rather than in those who consume meat, creatine supplementation resulted in better memory."

Planters and Meaters started out with the same memory abilities. Planters' memories improved when they took a creatine supplement; Meaters' didn't. So should Planters take supplements? Probably not, because of contamination with other unhealthy stuff.

Creatinine

Holland RD, Gehring T, Taylor J, Lake BG, Gooderham NJ, Turesky RJ. Formation of a mutagenic heterocyclic aromatic amine from creatinine in urine of meat eaters and vegetarians. *Chem. Res. Toxicol.* 2005 18(3):579–590.

"Creatinine and 2-aminobenzaldehyde are likely precursors of IQ[4,5-b]. The detection of IQ[4,5-b] in the urine of both meat eaters and vegetarians suggests that this HAA may be present in nonmeat staples or that IQ[4,5-b] formation may occur endogenously within the urinary bladder or other biological fluids."

Or it may be because vegetarians eat things that vegans don't, such as eggs, dairy and fishes, all of which can contain heterocyclic amines. (Why do researchers waste their time and energy on studying vegetarians?)

Diabetogens

PT Fujiyoshi, JE Michalek, F Matsumura. Molecular epidemiologic evidence for diabetogenic effects of dioxin exposure in U.S. Air force veterans of the Vietnam war. *Environ Health Perspect*. 2006 114(11):1677–1683.

Fujiyoshi et al found "a diabetogenic shift occurred in the biochemistry of adipose tissues from Vietnam veterans who were exposed to dioxin-containing Agent Orange herbicide preparations."

Thank you, Monsanto, for making diabolical chemicals and giving diabetes to Vietnam veterans and multitudes of others.

(Also in Monsanto's arsenal along with Agent Orange, Roundup and GM organisms are these devilish products - saccharin (beginning in1901), PCBs and bovine growth hormone. Maria Rodale writes in her excellent-for-a-doesn't-quite-get-it-Meater *Organic Manifesto*: "Every single one of the company's lines of business have wrought disaster, and yet it still survives and thrives."

And how bad must Monsanto's GM shit be if, as Rodale tells us, their CEO Hugh Grant told an interviewer in 2008 that he ate only organic food?)

Diacyl-glycerol

E W Kraegen, G J Cooney. Free fatty acids and skeletal muscle insulin resistance. *Curr Opin Lipidol*. 2008 Jun;19(3):235-41.

"Muscle lipid metabolites such as long chain fatty acid coenzyme As, diacylglycerol and ceramides may impair insulin signaling directly."

Saturated fats from animals and junk help cause diabetes.

Empty calories

Empty calories come from junk (and animals too.) The opposite concept is 'nutrient density.' Plants are high in nutrients, low in energy.

Sarter B, Campbell TC, Fuhrman J. Effect of a high nutrient density diet on long-term weight loss: a retrospective chart review. *Altern Ther Health Med*. 2008 May-Jun;14(3):48-53.

"An HND [high nutrient density, i.e. high-plant] diet… may be the most health-favorable and effective way to lose weight… Of the 19 patients who returned after 2 years, the mean weight loss was 53 lbs… , mean cholesterol fell by 13 points, LDL by 15 points, triglycerides by 17 points, and cardiac risk ratio dropped from 4.5 to 3.8. Changes in systolic and diastolic blood pressure were highly significant…"

We can choose how we lose weight: healthily with plants or unhealthily with lots of animals.

Endotoxins

Erridge C, Attina T, Spickett CM, Webb DJ. A high-fat meal induces low-grade endotoxemia: evidence of a novel mechanism of postprandial inflammation. *Am J Clin Nutr.* 2007 Nov; 86(5):1286-92.

"Bacterial endotoxin [lipopolysaccharide (LPS)], [is] a potently inflammatory bacterial antigen that is present in large quantities in the human gut… [There is]… increased circulating plasma endotoxin after a high-fat meal in healthy subjects. Increased postprandial LPS may contribute to the development of the postprandial inflammatory state, endothelial cell activation, and early events of atherosclerosis."

Dead bacteria or bacterial metabolites in the animals we eat cause after-meal inflammation and arterial "disease".

Endocrine disruptors (EDs)

Environmental hormone-disrupting chemicals enter our bodies mainly when we put the environment inside us: when we eat animals.

A. Bergman et al. The impact of endocrine disruption: A consensus statement on the state of the science. *Environ. Health Perspect.* 2013 121(4):A104-6.

"Many endocrine-related diseases and disorders are on the rise." The authors list

• low semen quality
• The incidence of genital malformations, such as non-descending testes (cryptorchidisms) and penile malformations (hypospadias), in baby boys
• The incidence of adverse pregnancy outcomes, such as preterm birth and low birth weight
• Neurobehavioral disorders associated with thyroid disruption

- [Increasing rates of] endocrine-related cancers (breast, endometrial, ovarian, prostate, testicular and thyroid)
- Earlier onset of breast development in young girls… a risk factor for breast cancer.
- [Dramatically increased] prevalence of obesity and type 2 diabetes… over the last 40 years.

Endocrine disruption's contribution to these disorders is a direct result of Meating.

Animal Estrogens

A Abrahamsson, V Morad, N M Saarinen, C Dabrosin. Estradiol, tamoxifen, and flaxseed alter IL-1β and IL-1Ra levels in normal human breast tissue in vivo. *J Clin Endocrinol Metab*. 2012 Nov;97(11):E2044-54.

"Sex steroid exposure increases the risk of breast cancer by unclear mechanisms. Diet modifications may be one breast cancer prevention strategy… The objective of this study was to elucidate whether estrogen, tamoxifen, and/or diet modification altered IL-1 levels in normal human breast tissue."

What did they find? Estrogens from animals cause breast cancer. Flax seeds (containing phyto-, or xenoestrogens) help combat breast cancer. As usual, Planting fixes what Meating causes.

Feces/Manure/Shit

J. L. W. Rademaker, M. M. M. Vissers, and M. C. T. Giffel. Effective heat inactivation of mycobacterium avium subsp. paratuberculosis in raw milk contaminated with naturally infected feces. *Appl. Environ. Microbiol.*, 73(13):4185-4190, 2007.

"High concentrations of feces from cows with clinical symptoms of Johne's disease were used to contaminate raw milk in order to realistically mimic possible incidents most closely."

You can't make this stuff up. Just so you're not missing the point here: to represent reality, these researchers took shit from sick cows and added it to milk.

Fish oil

There's evidence pro and con fish oil's role in the prevention of heart "disease" and cancer, largely on the basis of the long chain fatty acids DHA and EPA, with the most recent studies showing negative results. But what else is in fishes besides their fatty acids? Not anything good. Meaters say we should eat fishes for omega 3s is a bit like me saying Stalin was alright because he had a terrific moustache.

J M Ritchie et al. Organochlorines and risk of prostate cancer. J *Occup Environ Med.* 2003 Jul;45(7):692-702.

"…organochlorines… oxychlordane and PCB 180 were associated with an increased risk of prostate cancer."

That's the kind of stuff that's in fishes and the oils pressed from their dead bodies.

Free fatty acids
M Roden et al. Mechanism of free fatty acid-induced insulin resistance in humans. *J Clin Invest.* Jun 15, 1996; 97(12): 2859–2865.

Roden et al found that "that free fatty acids induce insulin resistance in humans by initial inhibition of glucose transport/phosphorylation which is then followed by an ~50% reduction in both the rate of muscle glycogen synthesis and glucose oxidation." Free fatty acids are a Meater issue.

Galactose
L A Batey et al. Skeletal health in adult patients with classic galactosemia. *Osteoporos Int.* 2013 Feb;24(2):501-9.

"Bone density in adults with galactosemia is low, indicating the potential for increased fracture risk."

If people with a genetic predisposition to high blood levels of this milk sugar have more osteoporosis, why would people who add dietary galactose also not be more osteoporotic? In fact, as we'll see under Osteoporosis later, milk drinkers are more prone to having brittle bones.

Gluten ~ Gliadin ~ Wheat protein
G De Palma et al. Effects of a gluten-free diet on gut microbiota and immune function in healthy adult human subjects. *Br J Nutr.* 2009 Oct;102(8):1154-60.

"… the GFD [gluten-free diet] led to reductions in beneficial gut bacteria populations and the ability of faecal samples to stimulate the host's immunity."

The tiny minority of people with celiac disease should avoid gluten because their lives depend on it. However, people without celiac disease are damaging their health by not eating gluten. As go our gut flora, so go we.

Harmane

E D Louis et al. Blood harmane, blood lead, and severity of hand tremor: Evidence of additive effects. *Neurotoxicology* 2011 32(2):227 – 232.

"Blood harmane and lead concentrations separately correlated with total tremor scores. Participants with high blood concentrations of both toxicants had the highest tremor scores, suggesting an additive effect of these toxicants on tremor severity."

That's why Essential Tremor is essentially a Meater condition: "Harmane (1-methyl-9H-pyrido[3,4-β]indole) is a potent β-carboline alkaloid [found] esp. in animal protein," and lead bioaccumulates in the fat of animals.

Heme iron

J C Fernandez-Cao et al. Heme iron intake and risk of new-onset diabetes in a Mediterranean population at high risk of cardiovascular disease: an observational cohort analysis. *BMC Public Health*. 2013 Nov 4;13:1042.

"The evidence examining the association between heme iron intake and CVD risk is limited to a few studies which suggest overall that high intakes of heme iron are associated with increased CVD risk. However it is possible that this could be due to other components of meat (the main source of heme iron) associated with CVD risk, such as saturated fats or other dietary and lifestyle factors associated with meat intake."

Well, okay then. It *may not* be the heme iron in animals that causes cardiovascular "disease"; it may be something else in the animals. Or something else as well as heme iron. Does it matter? Next time you order a steak, try asking your waitron to "hold the iron and the saturated fats and the animal proteins," see where that gets you.

Geoffrey C. Kabat, Thomas E. Rohan. Does excess iron play a role in breast carcinogenesis? an unresolved hypothesis. *Cancer Causes & Control* December 2007, Volume 18, Issue 10, pp. 1047-1053.

"In addition to its independent role as a pro-oxidant, high levels of free iron may potentiate the effects of estradiol, ethanol, and ionizing radiation— three established risk factors for breast cancer… Iron overload favors the production of reactive oxygen species, lipid peroxidation, and DNA damage, and may contribute to breast carcinogenesis..."

Heterocyclic amines (PhIP, MeIQx, IQ and IQ4,5b)

AE Norrish et al. Heterocyclic amine content of cooked meat and risk of prostate cancer. *J Natl Cancer Inst.* 1999 Dec 1; 91(23):2038-44.

"Meat doneness was weakly and inconsistently associated with prostate cancer risk for individual types of meat, but increased risk was observed for well-done beefsteak (relative risk = 1.68...)"

High Fructose Corn Syrup (HFCS)

George A Bray, Samara Joy Nielsen, and Barry M Popkin. Consumption of high-fructose corn syrup in beverages may play a role in the epidemic of obesity. *Am J Clin Nutr* 2004;79:537–43.

"It is becoming increasingly clear that soft drink consumption may be an important contributor to the epidemic of obesity, in part through the larger portion sizes of these beverages and through the increased intake of fructose from HFCS and sucrose."

The combination of meat + sweet is what fattens, sickens and kills us.

Homocysteine

S Seshadri et al. Plasma homocysteine as a risk factor for dementia and Alzheimer's disease. *N Engl J Med.* 2002 Feb 14;346(7):476-83.

M Hoffman. Hypothesis: hyperhomocysteinemia is an indicator of oxidant stress. *Med Hypotheses.* 2011 Dec;77(6):1088-93.

A H Ford, O P Almeida. Effect of homocysteine lowering treatment on cognitive function: a systematic review and meta-analysis of randomized controlled trials. *J Alzheimers Dis.* 2012;29(1):133-49.

Three papers that show the harms of Meating and the benefits of Planting.

Hydrogen sulfide

E Magee. A nutritional component to inflammatory bowel disease: the contribution of meat to fecal sulfide excretion. *Nutrition.* 1999 Mar;15(3):244-6.

"Dietary protein from meat is an important substrate for sulfide generation by bacteria in the human large intestine."

Animal protein is the very stuff meat is made from… and it's poisonous, because our gut flora turn it into a carcinogen. After millions of years of coexisting with us, our intestinal bacteria still don't like eating animals.

IGF-1 (Insulin-like growth factor-1)

M F McCarty. A low-fat, whole-food vegan diet, as well as other strategies that down-regulate IGF-1 activity, may slow the human aging process. *Med Hypotheses*. 2003 Jun;60(6):784-92.

"If down-regulation of IGF-I activity could indeed slow aging in humans, a range of practical measures for achieving this may be at hand. These include a low-fat, whole-food, vegan diet, exercise training, soluble fiber, insulin sensitizers, appetite suppressants, and agents such as flax lignans, oral estrogen, or tamoxifen that decrease hepatic synthesis of IGF-I. Many of these measures would also be expected to decrease risk for common age-related diseases."

Say no to the drugs and yes to the food. Animal proteins stimulate IGF-1 production and rapid cell division, leading to more cancer and faster aging.

Junk

R Moodie, D Stuckler, C Monteiro, N Sheron, B Neal, T Thamarangsi, P Lincoln, S Casswell, Lancet NCD Action Group. Profits and pandemics: prevention of harmful effects of tobacco, alcohol, and ultra-processed food and drink industries. *Lancet*. 2013 Feb 23;381(9867):670-9.

This is an extraordinary paper. Junk like salt and industrial sugar (sucrose) and corn syrup are three of the foremost (non-animal) killers in the industrial "food" supply.

"The 2011 UN high-level meeting on non-communicable diseases (NCDs) called for multisectoral action including with the private sector and industry. However, through the sale and promotion of tobacco, alcohol, and ultra-processed food and drink (unhealthy commodities), **transnational corporations are major drivers of global epidemics of NCDs**. What role then should these industries have in NCD prevention and control? We emphasise the rise in sales of these unhealthy commodities in low-income and middle-income countries, and consider the **common strategies that the transnational corporations use to undermine NCD prevention and control**. We assess the effectiveness of self-regulation, public–private partnerships, and public regulation models of interaction with these industries and conclude that **unhealthy commodity industries should**

have no role in the formation of national or international NCD policy. Despite the common reliance on industry self-regulation and public–private partnerships, there is no evidence of their effectiveness or safety. Public regulation and market intervention are the only evidence-based mechanisms to prevent harm caused by the unhealthy commodity industries." [Emphases added]

And get this – we don't often hear such courageous speaking of truth to power:

"In industrial epidemics, the vectors of spread are not biological agents, but transnational corporations. Unlike infectious disease epidemics, however, these **corporate disease vectors implement sophisticated campaigns to undermine public health interventions**. To minimise the harmful effects of unhealthy commodity industries on NCD prevention, we call for a substantially scaled up response from governments, public health organisations, and civil society to regulate the harmful activities of these industries."

Big "Food" and Big Chemical are lying us to death today just the way Big Smoke did for decades, and they're being abetted by their cronies in governmental, pharmaceutical and medical circles.

Lactose
PCRM. Understanding Lactose Intolerance.
www.pcrm.org/sites/default/files/pdfs/health/faq_lactintol.pdf

"Approximately 70 percent of African Americans, 90 percent of Asian Americans, 53 percent of Hispanic Americans, and 74 percent of Native Americans were lactose intolerant."

75% of the world's population cannot tolerate lactose. Consuming it leads to flatulence, constipation or diarrhea, at least.

LDL cholesterol
Spence JD. Fasting lipids: the carrot in the snowman. *Can J Cardiol.* 2003 Jul;19(8):890-2.

"Dietary cholesterol (one egg yolk), though it increases fasting low density lipoproteins by only about 10%, increases oxidized low-density lipoproteins by 34%... The current paradigm for the management of lipids is focused almost entirely on fasting lipid levels. However, most of the day is spent not in a fasting state, but in a postprandial [post-eating] state. Meals high in animal fat impair endothelial function for 4 hours... It is time to stop focusing only on fasting lipid levels and to begin paying more attention to outcomes."

How true. Measuring our cholesterol levels after a night's sleep, when most of the stuff has cleared our systems, gives artificially low readings. It's as if our water meter doesn't measure the amount we use after dark. Someone who thinks they're in the safe zone because their fasting LDL levels are "only" 100 may have real LDL levels much higher than that.

Methionine

B. C. Halpern, B. R. Clark, D. N. Hardy, R. M. Halpern, R. A. Smith. The effect of replacement of methionine by homocystine on survival of malignant and normal adult mammalian cells in culture. *Proc. Natl. Acad. Sci. USA* 1974 71(4):1133 - 1136.

In several cancers there is an "apparent absolute dependence of the malignant cells on preformed methionine," an amino acid found mainly in animals. "Absolute methionine dependence" is yet another good reason to be a pure Planter. We've known this for more than forty years.

Neu5Gc

Padler-Karavani V, Yu H, Cao H, Chokhawala H, Karp F, Varki N, Chen X, Varki A. Diversity in specificity, abundance, and composition of anti-Neu5Gc antibodies in normal humans: potential implications for disease. *Glycobiology*. 2008 Oct;18(10):818-30.

"As dietary Neu5Gc is primarily found in red meat and milk products, we suggest that this ongoing antigen-antibody reaction may generate chronic inflammation, possibly contributing to the high frequency of diet-related carcinomas and other diseases in humans."

This single animal component, which always causes a reaction from our immune system, is enough to disqualify animals as food.

Nitrites

Huncharek M, Kupelnick B. A meta-analysis of maternal cured meat consumption during pregnancy and the risk of childhood brain tumors. *Neuroepidemiology*. 2004 Jan-Apr;23(1-2):78-84.

"The data provide support for the suspected causal association between ingestion of NOCs [N-Nitroso compounds] from cured meats during pregnancy and subsequent CBT [childhood brain tumors] in offspring."

That's a long-winded, sciency way of saying that Meater mothers can give their babies cancer of the brain because of the nitrites in animals.

Nitrosamines and Nitrosamides/N-nitroso-compounds (NOCs)

N Ramirez, M Z Ozel, A C Lewis, R M Marce, F Borrull, J F Hamilton. Exposure to nitrosamines in third-hand tobacco smoke increases cancer risk in non-smokers. *Environ Int.* 2014 Oct;71:139-47.

"In addition to passive inhalation, non-smokers, and especially children, are exposed to residual tobacco smoke gases and particles that are deposited to surfaces and dust, known as third-hand smoke (THS)… The maximum risk from exposure to all nitrosamines measured in a smoker occupied home was one excess cancer case per one thousand population exposed. The results presented here highlight the potentially severe long-term consequences of THS exposure, particularly to children…"

If this is what nitrosamines do, why would we feed our kids hot dogs?

According to press release no. 240 of the WHO's International Agency for Research into Cancer on 26 October 2015, "Processed meat was classified as carcinogenic to humans (Group 1), based on sufficient evidence in humans that the consumption of processed meat causes colorectal cancer."

Cigarettes and animals are carcinogens. I'll say it again: Meating = Smoking.

PhIP

C. Wilson, A. Aboyade-Cole, O. Newell, E. Darling-Reed, E. Oriaku, R. Thomas. Diallyl sulfide inhibits PhIP-induced DNA strand breaks in normal human breast epithelial cells. *Oncology Reports* 2007 17(NA):807-811.

"Heterocyclic amines (HCAs) are formed when meat products such as beef, chicken, pork and fish are cooked at high temperatures. The most abundant HCA found in the human diet is 2-amino-1-methyl-6-phenylimidazo[4,5-b] pyridine (PhIP). PhIP… is associated with an increased risk of developing colon, breast, and prostate cancer … DAS inhibits PhIP-induced DNA strand breaks by inhibiting the production of reactive oxygen species. Therefore, we propose that DAS can prevent PhIP-induced breast cancer."

The PhIP in cooked flesh damages our DNA. Garlic prevents it. If we'd prefer not to have breast cancer, we should eat no animals and plenty of veggies, particularly alliums such as garlic, leeks and onions.

Phthalates

Meeker JD, Calafat AM, Hauser R. Urinary metabolites of di(2-ethylhexyl) phthalate are associated with decreased steroid hormone levels in adult men. *J Androl.* 2009 May-Jun;30(3):287-97.

"…urinary metabolites of DEHP [di(2-ethylhexyl) phthalate] are inversely associated with circulating steroid hormone levels in adult men."

Phthalates bioaccumulate in animals, and they're part of the reason why Meater men have lower testosterone levels than Planters. Phthalates can also lead to the feminization of male genitalia, or the 'undervirilization' of Meater males.

Phosphorus

R. A. Sherman, O. Mehta. Dietary phosphorus restriction in dialysis patients: Potential impact of processed meat, poultry, and fish products as protein sources. *Am. J. Kidney Dis.* 2009 54(1):18 - 23.

"Dietary intake of phosphorus is derived largely from protein [i.e. animal] sources and is a critical determinant of phosphorus balance in patients with chronic kidney disease."

R. A. Sherman, O. Mehta. Phosphorus and potassium content of enhanced meat and poultry products: Implications for patients who receive dialysis. *Clin J Am Soc Nephrol* 2009 4(8):1370 - 1373.

"The impact of addition of phosphorus to EMPP [enhanced meat and poultry products] is likely to be clinically significant, especially so in view of the probability that phosphorus in food additives is much better absorbed than phosphorus that is contained in unprocessed foods."

For healthy kidneys, we shouldn't eat animals. And then, if our kidneys are shot because we ate animals, we definitely shouldn't eat any more animals.

Polycyclic aromatic hydrocarbons (PAHs)

Chen JW, Wang SL, Hsieh DP, Yang HH, Lee HL. Carcinogenic potencies of polycyclic aromatic hydrocarbons for back-door neighbors of restaurants with cooking emissions. Sci Total Environ. 2012 Feb 15;417-418:68-75.

"In the present study, 21 polycyclic aromatic hydrocarbon (PAH) congeners were measured in the exhaust stack of 3 types of restaurants: 9 Chinese, 7 Western, and 4 barbeque (BBQ)…The total benzo[a]pyrene… concentrations… were highest in Chinese restaurants…, followed by Western... and BBQ-type restaurants... We further developed a probabilistic risk model to assess the incremental lifetime cancer risk (ILCR) for people exposed to carcinogenic PAHs."

Just living down-wind from Meaters can kill us.

Purines

Y Zhang, C Chen, H Choi, C Chaisson, D Hunter, J Niu, T Neogi. Purine-rich foods intake and recurrent gout attacks. *Ann Rheum Dis* 2012 71(9):1448 – 1453.

"The study findings suggest that acute purine intake increases the risk of recurrent gout attacks by almost fivefold among gout patients. Avoiding or reducing amount of purine-rich foods intake, especially of animal origin, may help reduce the risk of gout attacks."

High-fructose corn syrup also causes gout. Cherries fix it.

Pus

P. C. B. Vianna, G. Mazal, M. V. Santos, H. M. A. Bolini, and M. L. Gigante. Microbial and sensory changes throughout the ripening of prato cheese made from milk with different levels of somatic cells. *J. Dairy Sci.*, 91(5):1743-1750, 2008.

"The lower overall acceptance of the cheeses from high-SCC [somatic cell count; pus] milk may be associated with texture and flavor defect…"

Strange, that: people found that low-pus cheese tastes better.

Salt/sodium

He FJ, MacGregor GA. Effect of modest salt reduction on blood pressure: a meta-analysis of randomized trials. Implications for public health. *J Hum Hypertens.* 2002; 16:761–770.

"This meta-analysis strongly supports other evidence for a modest and long-term reduction in population salt intake, and would be predicted to reduce stroke deaths immediately by approximately 14% and coronary deaths by approximately 9% in hypertensives, and reduce stroke and coronary deaths by approximately 6 and approximately 4%, in normotensives, respectively."

The manufacturers of a drug this effective would own the world.

Steroids ~ sex hormones

L Aksglaede et al. The sensitivity of the child to sex steroids: possible impact of exogenous estrogens. *Hum Reprod Update*. 2006 Jul-Aug;12(4):341-9.

"Disrupted sex hormone action is… believed to be involved in the increased occurrence of genital abnormalities among newborn boys and precocious puberty in girls… Because no lower threshold for estrogenic action has been established, caution should be taken to avoid unnecessary exposure of fetuses and children to exogenous sex steroids and endocrine disruptors, even at very low levels."

In other words, pregnant mothers and their children shouldn't eat any animals at all.

TMA and TMAO

WHW Tang et al. Intestinal Microbial Metabolism of Phosphatidylcholine and Cardiovascular Risk. *N Engl J Med* 2013; 368:1575-1584.

"The production of TMAO from dietary phosphatidylcholine is dependent on metabolism by the intestinal microbiota. Increased TMAO levels are associated with an increased risk of incident major adverse cardiovascular events."

If we like eating eggs, we better enjoy them a whole lot because the choline in them increases our risk of heart attack, stroke and death.

The un-credible, indelible chemical egg.

Sidebar: Bacon and eggs - Eggs Bernays?

Edward Bernays, nephew of Sigmund Freud, the "Father of public relations" and author of *Propaganda* and *Crystallizing Public Opinion*, invented the dish we know as "bacon and eggs" in the 1920s to boost sales of bacon for the Beech-Nut Packing Company. Bernays co-opted "White Coat" "third party authorities" to say that "a heavy breakfast was sounder from the standpoint of health." (He tells the story, with no small self-satisfaction, at https://www.youtube.com/watch?v=KLudEZpMjKU.)

Ad slogans such as "4500 physicians urge bigger breakfast" [including bacon and eggs] sound eerily like the "More doctors smoke Camels than any other cigarette" jingle that would later help maim and kill millions more through lung cancer.

Apparently the devil takes care of his own. This highly influential, repugnant human being died in 1995, aged 103.

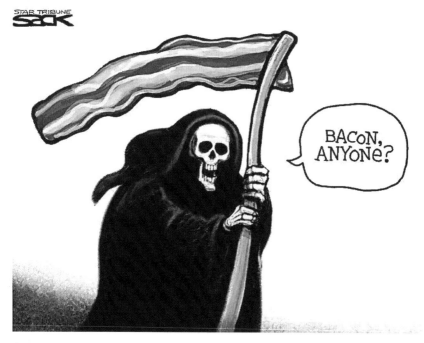

Cartoon, "Processed meat," thanks to Steve Sack, Star Tribune, 27 October 2015, following the WHO's announcement on the previous day that bacon and other processed meats are Group 1 carcinogens.

References to papers on "diseases" Meating causes

Acne
Loren Cordain, PhD; Staffan Lindeberg, MD, PhD, Magdalena Hurtado, PhD, Kim Hill, PhD, S. Boyd Eaton, MD and Jennie Brand-Miller, PhD. Acne Vulgaris: A Disease of Western Civilization. *Arch Dermatol* 2002,138:1584-1590.

"It is possible that low-glycemic diets may have therapeutic potential in reducing the symptoms of acne, a disease virtually unknown to the Aché and Kitavans."

Acne barely exists amongst people who don't eat lots of animals and junk… trust paleofantasist Cordain to emphasize the latter.

B Melnik. Milk consumption: Aggravating factor of acne and promoter of chronic diseases of western societies. *J Dtsch Dermatol Ges*, 7(4):364-370, 2009.

If the reader remembers just one fact from this book, there are few better than this: Acne = heart "disease" = cancer = hypertension = diabetes. They're all manifestations of the same thing: Meating and Junking.

In this brilliant paper, Bodo Melnik writes: "Milk is a complex fluid that developed over the course of mammalian evolution. Its primary function is to support growth and cell proliferation… Consumption of cow's milk and cow's milk protein result in changes of the hormonal axis of insulin, growth hormone and insulin-like growth factor-1(IGF-1) in humans."

These are not good things, and food shouldn't do them unless we're infants drinking our mother's breast milk.

"The epidemic incidence of adolescent acne in Western milk-consuming societies can be explained by the increased insulin- and IGF-1-stimulation of sebaceous glands mediated by milk consumption. Acne can be regarded as a model for chronic Western diseases with pathologically increased IGF-1-stimulation," which is also one of the pathways of cancer formation. We do *not* need alien hormones sloshing around in us and bossing us around.

Aggression
B. A. Golomb, M. A. Evans, H. L. White, J. E. Dimsdale. Trans fat consumption and aggression. *PLoS ONE* 2012 7(3):e32175

"Dietary trans fatty acids (dTFA) are primarily synthetic compounds that have been introduced only recently… Greater dTFA were strongly significantly associated with greater aggression, with dTFA more consistently predictive than other assessed aggression [and irritability] predictors… If the association is causal, the findings provide one further potential explanation for the recognized association between hostile/aggressive behaviors and heart disease. Trans fats could serve as common cause for both outcomes."

Trans fats are found in animals and junk, not in whole plants. Meating and junking make us irritable and aggressive.

Aging

D Ornish, J Lin, J Daubenmier, G Weidner, E Epel, C Kemp, M J M Magbanua, R Marlin, L Yglecias, P R Carroll, E H Blackburn. Increased telomerase activity and comprehensive lifestyle changes: a pilot study. *Lancet Oncol.* 2008 Nov;9(11):1048-57.

Dean Ornish does it yet again: first Planting conquered heart "disease" (1990), then prostate cancer (2005) and now it slows down cellular aging (2008), by increasing the length of our telomeres, the caps of our chromosomes. And that's great because:

"Telomere shortness in humans is emerging as a prognostic marker of disease risk, progression, and premature mortality. The aspect of cellular ageing that is conferred by diminished telomere maintenance seems to be an important precursor to the development of many types of cancer. Shortened telomeres predict poor clinical outcomes, including increased risk of metastasis in patients with breast cancer, increased risk of bladder, head and neck, lung, and renal-cell cancers, worse progression and prognosis of patients with colorectal cancer, prostate-cancer recurrence in patients undergoing radical prostatectomy, and decreased survival in patients with coronary heart disease and infectious disease."

Alzheimer's "disease"

Neal D. Barnard et al. Dietary and lifestyle guidelines for the prevention of Alzheimer's disease. *Neurobiology of Aging* 35 (2014) S74-S78.

Seven guidelines for the prevention of Alzheimer's emerged from The International Conference on Nutrition and the Brain, Washington, DC, July 19-20, 2013. The first two are:

"1. Minimize your intake of saturated fats and trans fats. Saturated fat is found primarily in dairy products, meats, and certain oils (coconut and palm oils). Trans fats are found in many snack pastries and fried foods and are listed on labels as "partially hydrogenated oils.""

In other words, no Meating or Junking.

"2. Vegetables, legumes (beans, peas, and lentils), fruits, and whole grains should replace meats and dairy products as primary staples of the diet."

In other words, whole Planting.

I guess none of the blithering idiots at the 'Nutrition and the Brain' conference bought Dr. David Perlmutter's idiotic, best-selling *Grain Brain*.

Amputations and Gangrene

MG Crane & C Sample. Regression of Diabetic Neuropathy with Total Vegetarian (Vegan) Diet. *Journal of Nutritional Medicine* Volume 4, Issue 4, 1994, pages 431-439.

Let's talk about diabetic neuropathy, the destruction of our peripheral or distal nerves in our limbs, which is the main cause of amputations. The authors speak of "systemic distal polyneuropathy (SDPN)."

On a Total Vegetarian Diet (TVD) – a vegan diet high in fiber and low in fat - plus exercise:

"Complete relief of the SDPN pain occurred in 17 of the 21 patients in 4 to 16 days… Follow-up studies of 17 of the 21 patients for 1-4 years indicated that 71% had remained on the diet and exercise programme as advised in nearly every item. In all except one of the 17 patients, the relief from the SDPN had continued, or there was further improvement."

These patients' blood glucose was "under good control [from] about the 10th day." When the diabetes goes away, the nerve damage goes away, and so does the risk of amputations. Planting does it routinely.

Angina

Göran K. Hansson and Peter Libby. The immune response in atherosclerosis: a double-edged sword. *Nature Reviews Immunology* volume 6 July 2006; 508-519.

"Although thrombi [blood clots] cause most of the acute complications of atherosclerosis, the gradual formation of stenoses [narrowings] that impede blood flow causes many of the chronic symptoms of atherosclerotic disease, such as angina pectoris (chest discomfort precipitated typically by physical or emotional stress)."

The authors call angina a "reversible attack of chest discomfort." It's permanently reversible on a Planter diet.

Asthma

L G Wood et al. Manipulating antioxidant intake in asthma: A randomized controlled trial. *Am J Clin Nutr.* 2012 96(3):534-543.

"Modifying the dietary intake of carotenoids alters clinical asthma outcomes. Improvements were evident only after increased fruit and vegetable intake, which suggests that whole-food interventions are most effective."

Whole plants help asthma sufferers; not animals, not junk, not supplements.

Atherosclerosis

W. C. Roberts. The cause of atherosclerosis. *Nutr Clin Pract,* 23(5):464-467, 2008.

"In summary, the connection between cholesterol elevation and atherosclerotic plaques is clear and well established. Atherosclerosis is a cholesterol problem! If one has elevated cholesterol, has an elevated blood pressure, smokes cigarettes, or has an elevated blood sugar, these additional factors serve to amplify the cholesterol damage but they by themselves do not produce atherosclerotic plaques! Societies with a high frequency of systemic hypertension or a high frequency of cigarette smoking but low cholesterol levels rarely get atherosclerosis."

As Roberts writes elsewhere, "It's the cholesterol, stupid." [http://www.ncbi.nlm.nih.gov/pmc/articles/PMC3012294/]

"No one has produced atherosclerosis experimentally by increasing the arterial blood pressure or glucose levels or by blowing smoke in the faces of rabbits their entire lifetime or by stressing these animals. The only way to produce atherosclerosis experimentally is by feeding high-cholesterol and/or high-saturated-fat diets to herbivores."

Roberts has been Editor–in–Chief of *The American Journal of Cardiology* since 1982.

Birth defects

S. J. Genuis. Nowhere to hide: Chemical toxicants and the unborn child. *Reprod. Toxicol.,* 28(1):115-116, 2009.

"…maternal exposure to toxic chemical compounds may be associated with various congenital defects, pediatric problems, skewed gender ratios, lethal cancers in children and teens, psychosexual challenges, as well as reproductive and endocrine dysfunction in later life. Just as endogenous hormones such as insulin, testosterone or estrogen have physiological or developmental effects at parts per billion, toxicants can also exert bioactive influence at exceedingly low levels."

In particular, "Gestational consumption of contaminated seafood remains a potential source of toxicant exposure, including mercury, for the developing child."

Dioxins, PCBs, DDT, heavy metals… I've devoted an entire section of this book to showing that the chemicals that cause birth defects and developmental disorders enter our bodies almost entirely through the animals we eat, mostly the fishes.

And if anyone's going to continue with the nonsense that we need to eat fishes to 'get' omega-3 fatty acids, please consider this study:

AW Turunen et al. Dioxins, polychlorinated biphenyls, methyl mercury and omega-3 polyunsaturated fatty acids as biomarkers of fish consumption. *Eur J Clin Nutr*, 64(3):313-323, 2010.

A biomarker is something we can measure that gives us a good idea about something else, which we usually can't measure as easily. In this study, Turunen et al present us with different ways of telling how many fishes someone eats. Now, if we measure our blood levels of omega-3s, that should be a good biomarker of fish consumption, right? Fishes are touted as a good source of omega-3s. The only problem with this is that there are better biomarkers for fish consumption: the toxic chemicals fishes have bio-accumulated in their flesh which we then bio-accumulate when we predate upon them.

"According to multiple regression modeling and LMG metrics, the most important fish consumption biomarkers were **dioxins** and **PCBs** among the men and **MeHg** [methyl mercury] among the women… Environmental contaminants seemed to be slightly better fish consumption biomarkers than omega-3 PUFAs in the Baltic Sea area."

It's no use eating fishes – even wild fishes – for the supposed benefits of their fats when their fats are so contaminated with chemical pollutants which more than undo the purported benefits of eating omega-3s.

Fishes aren't food, not even if one of their ingredients is supposedly beneficial. "Food is a package deal" and lethal pollutants are now an unavoidable part of the fish package.

Perhaps when the people at the Mayo Clinic get around to reading the Turunen paper, they'll remove salmon from their list of Top 10 Healthy Foods - Why They Are Good For You (Mayo Clinic News 1 August 2006).

Of salmon they say: "This fish is an excellent source of omega-3 fatty acids, which are believed to provide heart benefits. Salmon is also low in saturated fat and cholesterol and is a good source of protein. If possible, choose wild salmon, which is less likely to contain unwanted chemicals such as mercury."

Pretty much utter bollocks – 20th Century nutrition thinking. There is no safe lower intake of saturated fats or cholesterol (or mercury – not for our kids' brains.)

We'd all be better off eating the remaining 9 real foods on the Mayo list, though why they say wheat bran and vegetable juice instead of whole grains and whole vegetables is beyond me: Apples, Almonds, Broccoli, Blueberries, Red beans, Spinach, Sweet potatoes, Vegetable juice, Wheat germ.

Body odor
J. Havlicek and P. Lenochova. The effect of meat consumption on body odor attractiveness. *Chem. Senses* 31(8):747-752, 2006.

"Results of repeated measures analysis of variance showed that the odor of donors when on the nonmeat diet was judged as significantly more attractive, more pleasant, and less intense. This suggests that red meat consumption has a negative impact on perceived body odor hedonicity."

Without knowing it, Meaters smell bad. (There's a metaphor in there.)

Breast cancer
BJ Grube et al. White button mushroom phytochemicals inhibit aromatase activity and breast cancer cell proliferation. *J Nutr.* 2001 Dec;131(12):3288-93.

"Estrogen is a major factor in the development of breast cancer... diets high in mushrooms may modulate the aromatase activity and function in chemoprevention in postmenopausal women by reducing the in situ production of estrogen."

S. Choudhary, S. Sood, R. L. Donnell, H.-C. R. Wang. Intervention of human breast cell carcinogenesis chronically induced by 2-amino-1-methyl-6-phenylimidazo[4,5-b]pyridine. *Carcinogenesis* 2012 33(4):876 - 885

"More than 85% of breast cancers are sporadic and attributable to long-term exposure to environmental carcinogens, such as those in the diet, through a multistep disease process progressing from non-cancerous to premalignant and malignant stages. The chemical carcinogen 2-amino-1-methyl-6-phenylimidazo[4,5-b]pyridine (PhIP) is one of the most abundant heterocyclic amines found in high-temperature cooked meats and is recognized as a mammary carcinogen."

PhIP provides just one of the many Meater mechanisms of breast cancer.

Breast cancer healed or prevented

BR Goldin et al. Estrogen excretion patterns and plasma levels in vegetarian and omnivorous women. *N Engl J Med.* 1982 Dec 16;307(25):1542-7.

"We conclude that vegetarian women have an increased fecal output, which leads to increased fecal excretion of estrogen and a decreased plasma concentration of estrogen."

Planter women get less breast cancer because we out-poop our Meater sisters.

Adams LS, Chen S. Phytochemicals for breast cancer prevention by targeting aromatase. *Front Biosci.* 2009 Jan 1;14:3846-63.

Adams et al "discuss whole food extracts and the common classes of phytochemicals which have been investigated for potential aromatase inhibitory activity."

The isoflavones in soy exert a phytoestrogenic effect that counters animal estrogens. This is one probable reason why Asian women were free of breast cancer until their recent nutrition transition to Meating and Junking.

Cancer

D. Boivin et al. Antiproliferative and antioxidant activities of common vegetables: A comparative study. *Food Chem.*, 112(2):374-380, 2009.

"These results thus indicate that vegetables have very different inhibitory activities towards cancer cells and that **the inclusion of cruciferous and Allium vegetables in the diet is essential for effective dietary-based chemopreventive strategies**."

In other words, the broccoli and onion-&-garlic families prevent cancer.

Also: "…individuals who eat five servings or more of fruits and vegetables daily have approximately half the risk of developing a wide variety of cancer types, particularly those of the gastrointestinal tract."

EK Silbergeld, K Nachman. The environmental and public health risks associated with arsenical use in animal feeds. *Ann. N.Y. Acad. Sci.*, 1140:346-357, 2008.

"Arsenic exposures are among the most important environmental health risks in many regions of the world. Arsenic is a human carcinogen, and is also associated with increased risks of several noncancer endpoints, including cardiovascular disease, diabetes, neuropathy, and neurocognitive deficits in children."

Chickens and eggs are most contaminated, and it's added on purpose. But that's not all that's in chickens…

ES Johnson et al. Mortality from malignant diseases-update of the Baltimore union poultry cohort. *Cancer Causes Control*. 2010 Feb;21(2):215-21.

We've met the sad Baltimore union poultry cohort before. Johnson et al told us that oncogenic viruses in chickens are mainly responsible for their extraordinarily high cancer rates. "Other potentially carcinogenic occupational exposures include exposure to fumes emitted from the wrapping machine, nitrosamines during the curing of poultry, and to smoke or aerosol emitted during smoking or cooking of poultry products that contain polycyclic aromatic hydrocarbons and heterocyclic amines."

Animals themselves are poisonous; they contain other poisons; and cooking them creates still others.

"Compared to the US general population, an excess of cancers of the buccal and nasal cavities and pharynx (base of the tongue, palate and other unspecified mouth, tonsil and oropharynx, nasal cavity/middle ear/accessory sinus), esophagus, recto-sigmoid/rectum/anus, liver and intrabiliary system, myelofibrosis, lymphoid leukemia and multiple myeloma was observed in particular subgroups or in the entire poultry cohort. We hypothesize that oncogenic viruses present in poultry, and exposure to fumes, are candidates for an etiologic role to explain the excess occurrence of at least some of these cancers in the poultry workers."

If we eat poultry, we can add penis cancer to the list.

Collins AR, Harrington V, Drew J, Melvin R. Nutritional modulation of DNA repair in a human intervention study. *Carcinogenesis*. 2003 Mar; 24(3):511-5.

"Kiwifruit provides a dual protection against oxidative DNA damage, enhancing antioxidant levels and stimulating DNA repair. It is probable that together these effects would decrease the risk of mutagenic changes leading to cancer."

Kiwifruits are not alone among plants that provide this dual protection against cancer.

S Rohrmann et al. Consumption of meat and dairy and lymphoma risk in the European Prospective Investigation into Cancer and Nutrition. *Int J Cancer*. 2011 Feb 1;128(3):623-34.

In the EPIC study, Rohrmann et al found "that men and women with a high consumption of processed meat are at increased risk of early death, in particular due to cardiovascular diseases but also to cancer. In this population, reduction of processed meat consumption to less than 20 g/day would prevent more than 3% of all deaths."

In the USA, that would translate into about 75,000 fewer deaths each year... just from cutting out deli meats.

Loh YH, Jakszyn P, Luben RN, Mulligan AA, Mitrou PN, Khaw KT. N-Nitroso compounds and cancer incidence: the European Prospective Investigation into Cancer and Nutrition (EPIC)-Norfolk Study. *Am J Clin Nutr*. 2011 May;93(5):1053-61. Epub 2011 Mar 23.

N-nitroso compounds, or nitrosamines, are carcinogens found in animals, particularly highly processed animals, and cigarette smoke.

"Dietary [nitrosamines (NDMA) [N-nitrosodimethylamine] was associated with a higher gastrointestinal cancer incidence, specifically of rectal cancer."

Got meat? Got smoking? Got cancer of the butt.

This is the third time I'm saying this: Meating = Smoking.

Cardiovascular "disease"

SK Park et al. Fruit, vegetable, and fish consumption and heart rate variability: The veterans administration normative aging study. *Am. J. Clin. Nutr.*, 89(3):778-786, 2009.

"Conclusion: These findings suggest that higher intake of green leafy vegetables may reduce the risk of cardiovascular disease through favorable changes in cardiac autonomic function."

In other words, green leafy vegetables help keep our hearts beating.

JD Spence, DJ Jenkins, J Davignon. Dietary cholesterol and egg yolks: not for patients at risk of vascular disease. *J. Can J Cardiol.* 2010 Nov;26(9):e336-9.

"Dietary cholesterol, including egg yolks, is harmful to the arteries. Patients at risk of cardiovascular disease should limit their intake of cholesterol. Stopping the consumption of egg yolks after a stroke or myocardial infarction would be like quitting smoking after a diagnosis of lung cancer: a necessary action, but late. The evidence presented in the current review suggests that the widespread perception among the public and health care professionals that dietary cholesterol is benign is misplaced, and that improved education is needed to correct this misconception."

So, who's at risk of vascular "disease", according to Spence et al? Everyone who's eating the Standard American Diet of animals and junk.

Cataracts
PN Appleby, NE Allen, TJ Key. Diet, vegetarianism, and cataract risk. *Am J Clin Nutr.* 2011 May;93(5):1128-35.

"Vegetarians were at lower risk of cataract than were meat eaters in this cohort of health-conscious British residents."

Now imagine if they'd studied Planters.

Colon cancer ~ Colorectal cancer
O'Keefe SJ, Kidd M, Espitalier-Noel G, Owira P. Rarity of colon cancer in Africans is associated with low animal product consumption, not fiber. *Am J Gastroenterol.* 1999 May;94(5):1373-80.

"The low prevalence of colon cancer in black Africans cannot be explained by dietary "protective" factors, such as fiber, calcium, vitamins A, C and folic acid, but may be influenced by the absence of "aggressive" factors, such as excess animal protein and fat, and by differences in colonic bacterial fermentation."

When it comes to healthy outcomes of eating, it's either the good effects of Planting or the absence of the bad effects of Meating and Junking. The "differences in colonic bacterial fermentation" between cancer-provoking animal-fed gut flora and cancer-preventing, fiber-fed gut flora are immense.

Constipation

G Iacono et al. Intolerance of cow's milk and chronic constipation in children. *N Engl J Med*. 1998 Oct 15;339(16):1100-4.

Iacono et al tell us that "the concomitant presence of other manifestations of intolerance of cow's milk (**bronchospasm**, **dermatitis**, and **rhinitis**) increases the probability that constipation will be found to be a symptom of intolerance of cow's milk... clinical examination of the children in our study showed a very high frequency of severe **anal fissures**. Because these lesions reappeared after the reintroduction of cow's milk and before the onset of constipation, we hypothesize that they are one of the mechanisms causing constipation. **Pain on defecation** can cause retention of feces in the rectum, with consequent dehydration and hardening of the stools, thus aggravating constipation."

Does this muck sound like food? "Forty-four of the 65 children (68 percent) had a response while receiving soy milk." In other words, they got better when they stopped drinking cows' milk and started drinking plant milk – no more problems with breathing, skin conditions, hay fever, constipation or anal fissures.

Sanjoaquin MA, Appleby PN, Spencer EA, Key TJ. Nutrition and lifestyle in relation to bowel movement frequency: a cross-sectional study of 20630 men and women in EPIC-Oxford. *Public Health Nutr*. 2004 Feb;7(1):77-83.

"In conclusion, we have identified several nutritional and lifestyle factors that were associated with the frequency of bowel movements. The strongest associations were seen with having a vegetarian or vegan diet, dietary fibre intake, fluid intake and vigorous exercise."

Planters poop more often (and more) and, as a result, get sick less often and live longer. It's as basic as that. We shouldn't need any more information when deciding on a dietstyle.

COPD (chronic obstructive pulmonary "disease")

E Keranis et al. Impact of dietary shift to higher-antioxidant foods in COPD: a randomised trial. *Eur Respir J*. 2010 Oct;36(4):774-80.

"…a dietary shift to higher-antioxidant food intake may be associated with improvement in lung function, and, in this respect, dietary interventions might be considered in COPD management."

Plants are antioxidants; animals are oxidants – animals make it hard for people with emphysema to breathe.

Crohn's "disease"

C L Roberts et al. Translocation of Crohn's disease *Escherichia coli* across M-cells: contrasting effects of soluble plant fibres and emulsifiers. *Gut.* 2010 Oct;59(10):1331-9.

"Crohn's disease is common in developed nations where the typical diet is low in fibre and high in processed food… Translocation of *E coli* across M-cells is reduced by soluble plant fibres, particularly plantain and broccoli, but increased by the emulsifier Polysorbate-80."

Whole plant fibers ameliorate Crohn's "disease". Emulsifiers (such as dishwashing liquids and P-80 in junk) make matters worse.

Depression

M Berk et al. So depression is an inflammatory disease, but where does the inflammation come from? *BMC Med.* 2013 Sep 12;11:200.

"A range of factors appear to increase the risk for the development of depression, and seem to be associated with systemic inflammation; these include psychosocial stressors, poor diet, physical inactivity, obesity, smoking, altered gut permeability, atopy [allergies], dental cares, sleep and vitamin D deficiency. Most [of these] sources of inflammation may play a role in other psychiatric disorders, such as bipolar disorder, schizophrenia, autism and post-traumatic stress disorder."

Besides 'psychosocial stressors' ("Stuff happens"), Meating makes most depression factors worse, while Planting improves them. For example:

M E Payne et al. Fruit, vegetable, and antioxidant intakes are lower in older adults with depression. *J Acad Nutr Diet.* 2012 Dec;112(12):2022-7.

"These associations may partially explain the elevated risk of cardiovascular disease among older individuals with depression. In addition, these findings point to the importance of antioxidant food sources [i.e. whole plants] rather than dietary supplements."

Type 1 Diabetes

G. Dahlquist. The aetiology of type 1 diabetes: An epidemiological perspective. *Acta Paediatr Suppl.* 1998 425:5-10.

"Risk factors that may initiate the autoimmune process include early exposure to cow's milk proteins, nitrosamines or early foetal events such as blood group incompatibility or foetal viral infections."

There are no casein, nitrosamines or viruses in plants.

Type 2 Diabetes

M. A. Hyman, D. Ornish, M. Roizen. Lifestyle medicine: Treating the causes of disease. *Altern Ther Health Med* 2009 15(6):12 - 14.

"…the recent "EPIC" study published in the Archives of Internal Medicine studied 23 000 people's adherence to 4 simple behaviors (not smoking, exercising 3.5 hours a week, eating a healthy diet [fruits, vegetables, beans, whole grains, nuts, seeds, and limited amounts of meat], and maintaining a healthy weight [BMI <30]). In those adhering to these behaviors, 93% of diabetes, 81% of heart attacks, 50% of strokes, and 36% of all cancers were prevented."

Lifestyle medicine works better than any other medical intervention… and it's free. The authors conclude: "If lifestyle medicine becomes central to the practice of medicine, our sick care system will be transformed into a healthcare system."

A. Vang, P. N. Singh, J. W. Lee, E. H. Haddad, and C. H. Brinegar. Meats, processed meats, obesity, weight gain and occurrence of diabetes among adults: Findings from Adventist health studies. *Ann. Nutr. Metab.*, 52(2):96-104, 2008.

"Our findings raise the possibility that meat intake, particularly processed meats, is a dietary risk factor for diabetes."

So why does Dr. Mark Hyman promote animals-as-food? I have no idea.

Neal D Barnard, Heather I Katcher, David JA Jenkins, Joshua Cohen, and Gabrielle Turner-McGrievy. Vegetarian and vegan diets in type 2 diabetes management. *Nutrition Reviews*® Vol. 67(5):255–263.

According to Dr. Neal Barnard et al, "Several possible mechanisms may explain the effect of low-fat, plant-based diets on glycemic [sugar] control:

- Weight loss…
- Changes in intramyocellular lipid [fat inside muscle cells]…
- Reductions in saturated fat intake…
- Reduced glycemic index…
- Increased intake of dietary fiber…
- Reductions in iron stores."

Of the six mechanisms, low-carbers can provide weight loss and reduced glycemic load. Only Planting produces all six mechanisms for preventing diabetes. This is why many low-carbers remain or become diabetic even when they're skeletally thin on the outside: they're fiber-deficient and fat where it counts in nutrition – inside.

Planters have the best glycemic control, the least insulin resistance, the least diabetes and the fewest degenerative "diseases" overall.

WJ Crinnion. The role of persistent organic pollutants in the worldwide epidemic of type 2 diabetes mellitus and the possible connection to Farmed Atlantic Salmon (*Salmo salar*). *Altern Med Rev.* 2011 16(4):301 – 313.

"Recent studies reveal that the presence of several persistent organic pollutants (POPs) can confer greater risk for developing the disease than some of the established lifestyle risk factors [poor nutrition, obesity, lack of exercise]. In fact, evidence suggests the hypothesis that obesity might only be a significant risk factor when adipose tissue contains high amounts of POPs… Obesity is one of the most well-known risk factors associated with developing T2DM. The evidence on POPS and T2DM suggests that increased body fatness with low in vivo POPs levels does not place a person at increased risk, while increased adiposity with high levels of POPs does."

If this is true, it helps explain why Meaters have far worse insulin resistance and far more diabetes than Planters. It's partly because the animals they eat biomagnify POPs to obscene levels. As usual, carnivorous fishes such as salmons are the most contaminated.

And lastly, please note the title of the following paper – "Higher insulin sensitivity in vegans…"

J Gojda et al. Higher insulin sensitivity in vegans is not associated with higher mitochondrial density. *Eur J Clin Nutr.* 2013 Dec;67(12):1310-5.

I won't go into the details of this paper. What's important to grasp is that the baseline from which competent biomedical researchers work is this: Vegans have the highest insulin sensitivity, the least insulin resistance, and therefore the least diabetes. As usual, people on extremely high whole-carb diets have the best health outcomes.

Why more needs saying?

Gestational diabetes
C Qiu et al. Risk of gestational diabetes mellitus in relation to maternal egg and cholesterol intake. *Am. J. Epidemiol.* 2011 173(6):649 - 658.

"…high egg and cholesterol intakes before and during pregnancy are associated with increased risk of GDM [gestational diabetes mellitus]… relative risk… 2.52 for consumption of ≥10 eggs/week."

Diabetic retinopathy
N Cheung, P Mitchell, T Y Wong. Diabetic retinopathy. *Lancet.* 2010 Jul 10;376(9735):124-36.

"Optimum control of blood glucose, blood pressure, and possibly blood lipids remains the foundation for reduction of risk of retinopathy development and progression."

Who have the lowest blood glucose and cholesterol levels, and the lowest blood pressure? Planters. Who have the least diabetes and therefore the least diabetic retinopathy? Planters.

Diarrhea
X Xia et al. Presence and characterization of shiga toxin-producing *Escherichia coli* and other potentially diarrheagenic *E. coli* strains in retail meats. *Appl Environ Microbiol,* 76(6):1709-1717, 2010.

"…retail meats, mainly ground beef, were contaminated with diverse STEC strains."

Diarrheagenic bacteria such as *E. coli, C. diff* and *Y. enterocolitica* are animal-borne pathogens. No wonder Meaters get diarrhea so often.

Disc degeneration & herniation
U G Longo et al. Symptomatic disc herniation and serum lipid levels. *Eur Spine J.* 2011 Oct;20(10):1658-62.

"When comparing the two groups, patients with symptomatic herniated lumbar disc showed statistically significant higher triglyceride concentration... and total cholesterol concentration... Serum lipid levels may be a risk factor for IVD [intervertebral disc] pathology."

Meating damages the discs between the vertebrae of our spines.

Diverticulosis and Diverticulitis

NS Painter, DP Burkitt. Diverticular disease of the colon: a deficiency disease of Western civilization. *Br Med J*. 1971 May 22;2(5759):450-4.

Neil Painter and Denis Burkitt say: "We present a hypothesis as to the cause of diverticulosis coli which is consistent with its geographical distribution, its recent emergence as a medical problem, and its changing incidence.

Diverticulosis appears to be a deficiency disease caused by the refining of carbohydrates which entails the removal of vegetable fibre from the diet. Consequently we consider it to be preventable.

Diverticulitis first became a clinical problem at the turn of the century, and the term "diverticulosis" first appeared in 1914. As recently as 1916 the disease was not important enough to merit a mention in textbooks."

Both animals and junk are deficient or entirely lacking in fiber. Other consequences of fiber deficiency include constipation and all the resulting 'pressure diseases,' plus a host of other Western conditions.

Lisa L. Strate et al. Nut, Corn, and Popcorn Consumption and the Incidence of Diverticular Disease. *JAMA*. 2008;300(8):907-914.

"Patients with diverticular disease are frequently advised to avoid eating nuts, corn, popcorn, and seeds to reduce the risk of complications. However, there is little evidence to support this recommendation... In this large, prospective study of men without known diverticular disease, nut, corn, and popcorn consumption did not increase the risk of diverticulosis or diverticular complications. The recommendation to avoid these foods to prevent diverticular complications should be reconsidered."

Drug resistance

AE Waters et al. Multidrug-Resistant *Staphylococcus aureus* in US Meat and Poultry. *Clin Infect Dis*. 2011 May;52(10):1227-30.

"Conventional concentrated animal feeding operations (CAFOs) provide all the necessary components for the emergence and proliferation of multidrug-resistant zoonotic pathogens. In the United States, billions of food animals are raised in densely stocked CAFOs, where antibiotics are routinely administered in feed and water for extended periods to healthy animals. NARMS [the National Antimicrobial Resistance Monitoring System] has shown that multidrug-resistant *E. coli* and *Enterococcus* species are prevalent among US meat and poultry products. Our findings indicate that multidrug-resistant *S. aureus* should be added to the list of antimicrobial-resistant pathogens that routinely contaminate our food supply."

Eating animals is bringing us more infectious diseases, while simultaneously removing our ability to treat them.

Erectile dysfunction ~ Impotence

DR Meldrum et al. The link between erectile and cardiovascular health: The canary in the coal mine. *Am. J. Cardiol.* 2011 108(4):599-606.

I've said this a few times in different ways, but it bears saying again: Heart "disease" = acne = erectile dysfunction = lower back pain. They're all symptoms of Meating. If we have one, it's almost certain we have others, even if they're not yet clinically detectable.

"In men aged <60 years and in men with diabetes or hypertension, erectile dysfunction can be a critical warning sign for existing or impending cardiovascular disease and risk for death… by better understanding the complex factors influencing erectile and overall vascular health, physicians can help their patients prevent vascular disease and improve erectile function, which provides more immediate motivation for men to improve their lifestyle habits and cardiovascular health."

For men, passion is hydraulic, and Meating messes with our fluid pipes.

Fatty liver "disease"

There are two variants of fatter liver "disease" - alcoholic and nonalcoholic. What causes the latter, which now provides the majority of cases? Would you be surprised to hear 'Animals and Junk?'

A K Leamy, R A Egnatchik, J D Young. Molecular mechanisms and the role of saturated fatty acids in the progression of non-alcoholic fatty liver disease. *Prog Lipid Res.* 2013 Jan;52(1):165-74.

"…saturated fatty acids are more toxic than their unsaturated counterparts, resulting in a progressive lipotoxic cascade… fatty acid saturation plays a critical role in determining cell fate under lipotoxic conditions."

M K Hellerstein. Mitigating factors and metabolic mechanisms in fructose-induced nonalcoholic fatty liver disease: the next challenge. *Am J Clin Nutr.* 2012 Nov;96(5):951-2.

"Fructose homes in like a laser beam on the liver and its glycolytic pathways, with ~90% of fructose uptake by the liver. Fructose intake results in hepatic release of lactate, storage of glycogen, and stimulation of de novo fatty acid synthesis. Fructose shares this liver tropism with galactose [milk sugar], but perhaps a better analogy is ethanol. Like ethanol, fructose increases de novo lipogenesis (DNL), inhibits fatty acid oxidation, and has been implicated in NAFLD."

The 3 dietary villains in nonalcoholic fatty liver "disease"? Animal fats, animal sugar and junk sugar. Whole grains and oatmeal are protective.

Gallstones
Portincasa P, Moschetta A, Palasciano G. Cholesterol gallstone disease. *Lancet.* 2006 Jul 15;368(9531):230-9.

The title of this paper sums up gallstones: Cholesterol gallstone disease.

"Gallstones are abnormal masses of a solid mixture of cholesterol crystals, mucin, calcium bilirubinate, and proteins… In Western societies, cholesterol gallstones account for 80–90% of the gallstones found at cholecystectomy [surgical removal]. Precipitation of excess cholesterol in bile as solid crystals is a prerequisite for cholesterol gallstone formation."

And high levels of blood cholesterol (the result of eating saturated and trans fats and cholesterol) are a prerequisite for causing the "precipitation of excess cholesterol in bile as solid crystals" or stones in our gall bladders. Ouch. It's too bad that the agony of Meating is usually atopic and atemporal, occurring elsewhere and else-when, becoming evident only after years of eating non-meals.

Glaucoma
AL Coleman et al; Study of Osteoporotic Fractures Research Group. Glaucoma risk and the consumption of fruits and vegetables among older women in the study of osteoporotic fractures. *Am J Ophthalmol.* 2008 Jun;145(6):1081-9.

"A higher intake of certain fruits and vegetables may be associated with a decreased risk of glaucoma."

Gout

Under Purines earlier, Zhang et al told us we should avoid eating animals because of the purines they contain if we want to avoid gout.

Choi HK, Willett W, Curhan G. Fructose-rich beverages and risk of gout in women. *JAMA*. 2010 Nov 24;304(20):2270-8.

"Although sugar-sweetened beverages contain low levels of purine (i.e. the precursor of uric acid), they contain large amounts of fructose, which is the only carbohydrate known to increase uric acid levels."

Gout comes from animal purines and junk fructose, because they raise uric acid levels. As Falstaff says in 2 Henry IV: "A pox of this gout! or, a gout of this pox! For the one or the other plays the rogue with my great toe."

Think on Shakespeare's wordplay: Falstaff - fall staff - means erectile dysfunction, and ED = obesity = gout = stroke = heart "disease" etc.

Guillain-Barré syndrome

TA Hardy et al. Guillain-Barré syndrome: modern theories of etiology. *Curr Allergy Asthma Rep*. 2011 Jun;11(3):197-204.

"Guillain-Barré syndrome (GBS) is a classic failure of the immune system with a life-threatening attack upon a critical self-component... Triggers for GBS include infection... particularly [with] *Campylobacter jejuni*."

How do we become infected with *Campylobacter*?

Mainly by eating chickens.

Nachamkin I, Allos BM, Ho T. *Campylobacter* species and Guillain-Barré syndrome. *Clin Microbiol Rev*. 1998 Jul;11(3):555-67.

"*C. jejuni* is the most common cause of bacterial gastroenteritis in the United States, surpassing *Salmonella* in most studies. It is estimated that over 2.5 million cases occur each year in the United States."

'Playing chicken' takes on a new meaning when it comes to total paralysis.

Heart "disease" (Coronary artery "disease", Cardiac "disease")

W. F. Enos, R. H. Holmes, J. Beyer. Coronary disease among United States soldiers killed in action in Korea preliminary report. Journal of the American Medical Association 1953 152(12):1090 - 1093.

Back in the early 1950s, way, way, way before today's Low-Carb Bullshit Artists say we became fat and sick because of all the sugar we're eating, autopsied American soldiers in the Korean police action, with an average age of 22.1 years old, were found to be riddled with heart "disease". And it wasn't because of all the smoking they were doing. As the Japanese population used to prove, before their lethal transition to the SAD diet, high smoking rates allied with low animal-eating rates lead to low cancer and heart "disease" rates.

According to Enos et al: "In 77.3% of the hearts, some gross evidence of coronary arteriosclerosis was found. The disease process varied from "fibrous" thickening to large atheromatous plaques causing complete occlusion of one or more of the major vessels." At 22 years old.

Here's another oldie but goody: A. G. Shaper, K. W. Jones. Serum-cholesterol, diet, and coronary heart-disease in Africans and Asians in Uganda: 1959. *Int J Epidemiol*. 2012 41(5):1221-1225.

"In the African population of Uganda coronary heart disease is almost non-existent… In the Asian community, on the other hand, coronary heart disease is a major problem."

Interesting. What's going on here? Is it genetic? Or is it the food?

It's the food, with the healthy indigenous African population eating the following and staying heart attack-free:

"The staple foods, green plantain and sweet potatoes, are steamed in banana leaves; cassava, yams, maize, and millet are also staple commodities in particular of the non-Baganda groups, while pumpkins, tomatoes, and green leafy vegetables are taken by all. The adequacy of protein in the diet depends almost entirely on the extent to which pulses, groundnuts, and cereals are used. Most meals are served with a sauce made of groundnuts, beans, and a mixture of vegetables, and occasionally meat or fish, and these are fried in very small amounts of fat…" Sounds almost ideal.

Ornish D, Brown SE, Scherwitz LW, Billings JH, Armstrong WT, Ports TA, McLanahan SM, Kirkeeide RL, Brand RJ, Gould KL. Can lifestyle changes reverse coronary heart disease? The Lifestyle Heart Trial. *Lancet*. 1990 Jul 21;336(8708):129-33.

"Overall, 82% of experimental-group patients had an average change towards regression. Comprehensive lifestyle changes may be able to bring about regression of even severe coronary atherosclerosis after only 1 year, without use of lipid-lowering drugs."

Those two dry sentences changed the world, or should have... In just one year of Planting (+ relaxation and exercise and other desirable but non-essential lifestyle changes), four out of five patients' heart conditions improved. No drugs, no surgery... and Lifestyle Medicine was born.

That the entire medical community hasn't sat up and taken notice of this landmark of medical landmarks is a scandal that will resound down the ages.

Esselstyn CB Jr. Resolving the Coronary Artery Disease Epidemic Through Plant-Based Nutrition. *Prev Cardiol.* 2001 Autumn;4(4):171-177.

Another genius, confirming Ornish's work... Here's his opening paragraph:

"The world's advanced countries have easy access to plentiful high-fat food; ironically, it is this rich diet that produces atherosclerosis. In the world's poorer nations, many people subsist on a primarily plant-based diet, which is far healthier, especially in terms of heart disease. To treat coronary heart disease, a century of scientific investigation has produced a device-driven, risk factor-oriented strategy. Nevertheless, many patients treated with this approach experience progressive disability and death. This strategy is a rear-guard defensive one. In contrast, compelling data from nutritional studies, population surveys, and interventional studies support the effectiveness of a plant-based diet and aggressive lipid lowering to arrest, prevent, and selectively reverse heart disease. In essence, this is an offensive strategy. The single biggest step toward adopting this strategy would be to have United States dietary guidelines support a plant-based diet. An expert committee purged of industrial and political influence is required to assure that science is the basis for dietary recommendations."

Esselstyn concludes: "We are fortunate to possess the knowledge of how to prevent, arrest, and selectively reverse this disease. [Planting.] However, we are not fortunate in the capacity of our institutions to share this information with the public. The collective conscience and will of our profession is being tested as never before. Ties to industry and politics result in conflict within our private and governmental health institutions, compromising the accuracy of their public message. This is in total violation of the moral imperative of our profession. Now is the time for us to have the courage for legendary work. Science — not the messenger — must dictate the recommendations."

And, finally, a word from the man beloved of Low-Carb Bullshit Artists for his development of the Glycemic Index...

DJ Jenkins et al. The Garden of Eden – plant based diets, the genetic drive to conserve cholesterol and its implications for heart disease in the 21st century. *Comp Biochem Physiol A Mol Integr Physiol.* 2003 Sep;136(1):141-51.

"We conclude that reintroduction of plant food components, which would have been present in large quantities in the plant based diets eaten throughout most of human evolution into modern diets can correct the lipid abnormalities associated with contemporary eating patterns and reduce the need for pharmacological interventions."

In a short video called "Dr. David Jenkins discusses the glycemic index of foods," he says: The glycemic index "is a difficult horse to ride. You can be thrown off quite easily." Like me, Jenkins thinks low-carb and paleo diets are a load of horse feathers, and that low-carb cowboys are 'all hat, no cattle' greenhorns who can't stay astride the frisky GI pony.

Hemorrhoids

Denis P. Burkitt. Some Diseases Characteristic of Modern Western Civilization. *British Medical Journal*, 1973, 1, 274-278.

"A number of diseases of major importance are characteristic of modern Western civilization. These diseases are rare or unknown in communities who have deviated little from their traditional way of life, and a rise in their frequency follows adoption of Western customs... Haemorrhoids are believed to be present to some degree in nearly half of all people over the age of 50."

It's not just the fiber in the diet that prevents piles. It's many different phytonutrients working together in concert within a high-fiber diet.

Neither Meating nor Junking is a high-fiber diet.

Hiatus hernia

Continuing with Burkitt (1973, above):

"Hiatus Hernia and Faecal Arrest

The close epidemiological relationship between hiatus hernia and a low-residue diet could well be accounted for by the raised intra-abdominal

674

pressures consequent on such a diet. Constrictive clothing and adiposity have been considered to be causes of increased intra-abdominal pressures contributing to hiatus hernia, but these must cause insignificant pressure change compared with straining at stool."

Meating and Junking are constipating and cause the 'pressure diseases.'

Hyperactivity ~ ADHD (Attention Deficit Hyperactivity Disorder)

D McCann et al. Food additives and hyperactive behaviour in 3-year-old and 8/9-year-old children in the community: a randomised, double-blinded, placebo-controlled trial. *Lancet*, Vol 370, #9598, 1560 - 1567, 3 Nov 2007.

"Artificial colours or a sodium benzoate preservative (or both) in the diet result in increased hyperactivity in 3-year-old and 8/9-year-old children in the general population.**"**

Junk isn't food, so why do we feed it to our precious children?

Hypertension

F M Sacks, E H Kass. Low blood pressure in vegetarians: effects of specific foods and nutrients. *Am J Clin Nutr*. 1988 Sep;48(3 Suppl):795-800.

"Strict vegetarians, who eat little if any animal products and lactovegetarians, who regularly eat dairy products, have lower blood pressures than the general population… modest intake of animal products may be a marker for a large intake of other potentially beneficial nutrients from vegetable products."

Hey, this paper was written in 1988, so let's cut the authors some slack. A quarter century later, we can say that cutting out all animal products leads to normotension, i.e. normal blood pressure.

J Stamler et al; INTERMAP Research Group. Glutamic acid, the main dietary amino acid, and blood pressure: the INTERMAP Study. *Circulation*. 2009 Jul 21;120(3):221-8.

"Dietary glutamic acid may have independent BP lowering effects, possibly contributing to the inverse relation of vegetable protein to BP."

The more plants we eat, the lower our blood pressure. Flaxseeds are terrific at countering hypertension.

Hypertensive retinopathy

Walter Kempner, MD. Treatment of Hypertensive Vascular Disease with Rice Diet. *American Journal of Medicine* 1948 pp. 545-577.

"Vascular retinopathy has been found to disappear with the rice diet. The retinal improvement does not necessarily coincide with decrease in blood pressure. Very severe retinopathy has disappeared in patients when the blood pressure remained at a constant high level or showed only an insignificant reduction."

Tiny arteries in the eye may benefit from Planting way before systemic blood pressure comes down.

"Those patients in whom the retinopathy remained unchanged had been on the diet from one to three and one-half months except for one patient with exudative stippling who was on the rice diet for nineteen months. The patients in whom the retinopathy cleared up only partially had been on the rice diet from one to seventeen months, an average of five months. The period of time in which the retinal changes disappeared completely ranged from two to thirty months, an average of fourteen months."

Plants are powerful healers.

Iatrogenic deaths

J Lazarou et al. Incidence of adverse drug reactions in hospitalized patients: a meta-analysis of prospective studies. *JAMA*. 1998 Apr 15; 279(15):1200-5.

The objective was to "estimate the incidence of serious and fatal adverse drug reactions (ADRs) in hospital patients… We estimated that in 1994 overall 2 216 000 hospitalized patients had serious ADRs and 106 000 had fatal ADRs, making these reactions between the fourth and sixth leading cause of death."

And that's just deaths of people taking the correct on-prescription meds, prescribed by physicians… no medical errors or in-hospital infections.

Infectious "diseases"

D W Eyre et al. Diverse sources of *C. difficile* infection identified on whole-genome sequencing. *N Engl J Med*. 2013 Sep 26;369(13):1195-205.

"It has been thought that *Clostridium difficile* infection is transmitted predominantly within health care settings. However, endemic spread" is on the rise. "Over a 3-year period, 45% of *C. difficile* cases in Oxfordshire were genetically distinct from all previous cases."

In other words, 45% of *C. diff* infections are now spreading within the community at large.

Where are the bacteria coming from? They're in the "food" supply, particularly in the pigs we eat.

Why? Because of fecal contamination among densely packed pigs in farrowing crates and other situations in which animals are hyper-confined.

The same applies to a multitude of other animal-borne pathogens.

Infectobesity

Pasarica M, Dhurandhar NV. Infectobesity: obesity of infectious origin. *Adv Food Nutr Res.* 2007;52:61-102.

"Of the several etiological factors [of obesity], infection, an unusual causative factor, has recently started receiving greater attention. In the last two decades, 10 adipogenic pathogens were reported, including human and nonhuman viruses, scrapie agents, bacteria, and gut microflora."

Chickens are the main host of obesity-causing viruses, principally avian adenovirus SMAM-1.

Kidney failure

Lin J, Hu FB, Curhan GC. Associations of diet with albuminuria and kidney function decline. *Clin J Am Soc Nephrol.* 2010 May; 5(5):836-43.

"Higher dietary intake of animal fat and two or more servings per week of red meat may increase risk for microalbuminuria [protein in the urine, a sign of kidney failure]. Lower sodium and higher B-carotene intake may reduce risk for eGFR [Estimated Glomerular Filtration Rate] decline."

More animals + more junk = more decline in kidney function.

Kidney stones

C R Tracy, S Best, A Bagrodia, J R Poindexter, B Adams-Huet, K Sakhaee, N Maalouf, C Y Pak, M S Pearle. Animal protein and the risk of kidney stones: a comparative metabolic study of animal protein sources. J Urol. 2014 Jul;192(1):137-41.

"Consuming animal protein is associated with increased serum and urine uric acid in healthy individuals. The higher purine content of fish compared to beef or chicken is reflected in higher 24-hour urinary uric acid. However, as reflected in the saturation index, the stone forming propensity is marginally higher for beef compared to fish or chicken. Stone formers should be advised to limit the intake of all animal proteins, including fish."

Who forms kidney stones? People who eat animals. Meaters. So they should be advised not to eat animals.

MD Sorensen et al, Women's Health Initiative Writing Group. Dietary intake of fiber, fruit and vegetables decreases the risk of incident kidney stones in women: a Women's Health Initiative report. *J Urol.* 2014 Dec;192(6):1694-9.

What do you know? Planting can prevent kidney stones. Why? More of the good PLUS less of the bad:

"Greater intake of fruits, vegetables, and fiber likely contributes to decreased intake of foods that are high in calories, sodium, fat, and animal protein."

Lou Gehrig's "disease" ~ ALS ~ Amyotrophic Lateral Sclerosis

W Holtcamp. The Emerging Science of BMAA: Do Cyanobacteria Contribute to Neurodegenerative Disease? *Environ Health Perspect.* 2012 Mar; 120(3): a110–a116.

"In addition to protein misincorporation, high levels of unbound BMAA can continually overstimulate glutamate receptors on cells, leading to neuronal injury… **BMAA and methyl mercury** – a common pollutant in seafood – both **deplete glutathione**, the main endogenous antioxidant in the body, and they act synergistically to harm nerve cells."

β-Methylamino-L-alanine, or BMAA, is an amino acid that's made by blue-green algae and which then becomes concentrated in the fatty flesh of sea animals – fishes, oysters, mussels, crabs. And when we eat them, BMAA becomes concentrated in our fatty brains, and especially in the brains of people suffering from neurodegeneration, such as Alzheimer's and Parkinson's victims.

Macular degeneration

S. Beatty et al. Macular pigment and risk for age-related macular degeneration in subjects from a Northern European population. *Invest. Ophthalmol. Vis. Sci.* 2001 42(2):439 - 446.

"Human macular pigment (MP) consists of the two hydroxycarotenoids, lutein (L) and zeaxanthin (Z), with concentrations that peak at the center of the fovea. MP is an effective filter of damaging blue light, which causes photo-oxidative retinal injury… Further, L and Z are powerful antioxidants… Consequently, it has been hypothesized that MP protects against AMD [age-related macular degeneration]... The macular pigment is entirely of dietary origin..."

The macular pigment of our eyes is made entirely out of the plants we eat.

JM Stringham et al. The influence of dietary lutein and zeaxanthin on visual performance. *J Food Sci.* 2010 Jan-Feb;75(1):R24-9.

"...the [plant] pigments protect the retina and lens, and perhaps even help to prevent age-related eye diseases such as macular degeneration... and cataract."

L Ma et al. Lutein and zeaxanthin intake and the risk of age-related macular degeneration: A systematic review and meta-analysis. *Br. J. Nutr.* 2012 107(3):350 - 359.

"...an increase in the intake of these carotenoids may be protective against late AMD."

We need to eat lots of plants if we want to see well when we're old.

Metabolic syndrome

Rizzo NS, Sabaté J, Jaceldo-Siegl K, Fraser GE. Vegetarian dietary patterns are associated with a lower risk of metabolic syndrome: the Adventist health study 2. *Diabetes Care.* 2011 May;34(5):1225-7.

"A vegetarian dietary pattern is associated with a more favorable profile of MRFs [metabolic risk factors]... (HDL, triglycerides, glucose, blood pressure, and waist circumference)... and a lower risk of MetS [metabolic syndrome].

Mood

Beezhold BL, Johnston CS, Daigle DR. Preliminary evidence that vegetarian diet improves mood. American Public Health Association annual conference, November 7-11, 2009. Philadelphia, PA.

"An omnivorous diet is typically higher in fat and protein, and contains less healthy fatty acid proportions than vegetarian diets. Research has shown that these dietary factors can promote subtle but adverse changes in the brain that impair mood state...

FISH participants significantly increased their EPA/DHA intakes and decreased their saturated fat intake but mood scores were not significantly reduced.

Conclusion: The complete restriction of flesh foods significantly reduced mood variability in omnivores."

Arachidonic acid is a polyunsaturated omega-6 fatty acid found in animals that causes brain inflammation.

Beezhold BL, Johnston CS, Daigle DR. Vegetarian diets are associated with healthy mood states: a cross-sectional study in seventh day Adventist adults. *Nutr J.* 2010 Jun 1;9:26.

"Vegetarians reported significantly less negative emotion than omnivores… participants with low intakes of EPA, DHA, and AA and high intakes of ALA and LA had better mood.

Conclusions: The vegetarian diet profile does not appear to adversely affect mood despite low intake of long-chain omega-3 fatty acids."

Mortality ~ Death

If there's one thing that Meaters and Junkers are better at than Planters, it's dying. It's not fair: Meaters and Junkers get so much more practice.

R. Sinha et al. Meat intake and mortality: a prospective study of over half a million people. *Arch Intern Med.* 2009 March 23; 169(6): 562–571.

"Red and processed meat intakes were associated with modest increases in total mortality, cancer mortality and CVD mortality."

Meating kills, so my modest proposal for increased longevity is that we shouldn't eat animals.

P. N. Singh, J. Sabaté, and G. E. Fraser. Does low meat consumption increase life expectancy in humans? *American Journal of Clinical Nutrition*, 78(3):526, 2003.

"Current prospective cohort data from adults in North America and Europe raise the possibility that a lifestyle pattern that includes a very low meat intake is associated with greater longevity… a longer duration (≥ 2 decades) of adherence to this diet contributed to a significant decrease in mortality risk and a significant 3.6-year increase in life expectancy."

How much is 3.6 years of life worth to you? I guarantee you, when you're sucking your last gasp you'll be willing to give everything you own for 3.6 more minutes.

Baer HJ, Glynn RJ, Hu FB, Hankinson SE, Willett WC, Colditz GA, Stampfer M, Rosner B. Risk factors for mortality in the nurses' health study: a competing risks analysis. *Am J Epidemiol.* 2011 Feb 1; 173(3):319-29.

"Age, body mass index at age 18 years, weight change, height, current smoking and pack-years of smoking, glycemic load, cholesterol intake, systolic blood pressure and use of blood pressure medications, diabetes, parental myocardial infarction before age 60 years, and time since menopause were directly related to all-cause mortality, whereas there were inverse associations for physical activity and intakes of nuts, polyunsaturated fat, and cereal fiber."

Inverse associations means that being active and eating plants are associated with living longer lives. Meating, Junking, smoking, being older, taking medications and having bad genes are associated with dying sooner.

H. Noto, A. Goto, T. Tsujimoto, M. Noda. Low-carbohydrate diets and all-cause mortality: A systematic review and meta-analysis of observational studies. *PLoS ONE* 2013 8(1):e55030.

I cited this study earlier to show why hyper-Meaters die more often. Here's another quote from Noto et al:

"…low-carbohydrate diets tend to result in reduced intake of fiber and fruits, and increased intake of protein from animal sources, cholesterol and saturated fat, all of which are risk factors for mortality and CVD [cardiovascular disease]… Our meta-analysis supported long-term harm and no cardiovascular protection with low-carbohydrate diets."

Why would one bother with questionable low-carb diets when there is no question about the long-term benefits of whole-food veganism?

How important is it to eat fruits and vegetables?

A Bellavia et al. Fruit and vegetable consumption and all-cause mortality: A dose-response analysis. *Am J Clin Nutr.* 2013 98(2):454 – 459.

"In comparison with 5 servings FV/d [fruits and vegetables per day], a lower consumption was progressively associated with shorter survival and higher mortality rates. Those who never consumed FV lived 3 y shorter… and had a 53% higher mortality rate… than did those who consumed 5 servings FV/d. Consideration of fruit and vegetables separately showed that those who never consumed fruit lived 19 mo shorter… than did those who ate 1 fruit/d. Participants who consumed 3 vegetables/d lived 32 mo longer than did those who never consumed vegetables…

Conclusion: FV consumption <5 servings/d is associated with progressively shorter survival and higher mortality rates."

There's a dose-response between added fruits and vegetables and extra years of life. This finding was confirmed by the massive Global Burden of Disease study, funded by the Bill and Melinda Gates Foundation, but in the negative: the biggest killer on planet Earth may be **not eating enough fruits and vegetables**, responsible for 4.9 million deaths around the world each year. Who doesn't eat enough whole plants? Junkers, poor people, and wealthy low-carb/paleo twits.

R Lozano et al. Global and regional mortality from 235 causes of death for 20 age groups in 1990 and 2010: a systematic analysis for the Global Burden of Disease Study 2010. *The Lancet.* Volume 380, No. 9859, p2095–2128, 15 December 2012.

"…dietary risk factors and physical inactivity were responsible for the largest disease burden… in 2010. Of the individual dietary risk factors, the largest attributable burden in 2010 was associated with diets **low in fruits** (4·9 million… deaths… followed by diets **high in sodium** (4·0 million…), **low in nuts and seeds** (2·5 million…), **low in whole grains** (1·7 million…), **low in vegetables** (1·8 million…), and **low in seafood omega-3 fatty acids** (1·4 million…)"

I think they're out to lunch about seafood omega-3s, because if we were all Planters almost no one would die of an omega deficiency, but let's not quibble. Most deaths are caused by plant deficiencies – 10.9 million people – followed by high-Junk diets.

More than 14.9 million of us humans die each year because we're not whole-food vegans.

Mucus production
Bartley J, McGlashan SR. Does milk increase mucus production? *Medical Hypotheses.* 2010 Apr;74(4):732-4.

Yes, for many: "a subgroup of the population, who have increased respiratory tract mucus production, find that many of their symptoms, including asthma, improve on a dairy elimination diet."

Multiple sclerosis

R. L. Swank, B. B. Dugan. Effect of low saturated fat diet in early and late cases of multiple sclerosis. *Lancet* 1990 336(8706):37-39.

"144 multiple sclerosis patients took a low-fat diet for 34 years. For each of three categories of neurological disability (minimum, moderate, severe) patients who adhered to the prescribed diet (≤20 g fat/day) showed significantly less deterioration and much lower death rates than did those who consumed more fat than prescribed (>20 g fat/day). The greatest benefit was seen in those with minimum disability at the start of the trial; in this group, when those who died from non-MS diseases were excluded from the analysis, 95% survived and remained physically active."

Since Dr. Roy Laver Swank started publishing his findings about the healing power of whole plants for sufferers of MS, such as "Multiple sclerosis: a correlation of its incidence with dietary fat," in *The American journal of the medical sciences* (1950), there has been no better treatment found. Dr. John McDougall continues his pioneering work today. My best guess is that his cutting out the fishes and fish oils Swank allowed will lead to improved results. It's too soon to tell.

Obesity

Rosell M, Appleby P, Spencer E, Key T. Weight gain over 5 years in 21,966 meat-eating, fish-eating, vegetarian, and vegan men and women in EPIC-Oxford. *Int J Obes* (Lond). 2006 Sep;30(9):1389-96.

"Men and women who changed their diet in one or several steps in the direction meat-eater → fish-eater → vegetarian → vegan showed the smallest mean annual weight gain of 242… and 301 g, respectively… During 5 years follow-up, the mean annual weight gain in a health-conscious cohort in the UK was approximately 400 g. Small differences in weight gain were observed between meat-eaters, fish-eaters, vegetarians and vegans. Lowest weight gain was seen among those who, during follow-up, had changed to a diet containing fewer animal foods."

We saw this earlier with the studies of 7th Day Adventists: vegans weigh substantially less and get less diabetes, hypertension – you name it – and live years longer:

S. Tonstad, T. Butler, R. Yan, and G. E. Fraser. Type of vegetarian diet, body weight, and prevalence of type 2 diabetes. *Diabetes Care*, 32(5). 791-796, 2009.

"Mean BMI was lowest in vegans (23.6 kg/m²) and incrementally higher in lacto-ovo-vegetarians (25.7 kg/m²), pesco-vegetarians (26.3 kg/m²), semi-vegetarians (27.3 kg/m²), and nonvegetarians (28.8 kg/m²)... The 5-unit BMI difference between vegans and nonvegetarians indicates a substantial potential of vegetarianism to protect against obesity." [I think scientists compete for the driest tone while announcing startling findings.]

Any diet book that doesn't mention how whole-food veganism is the best weight maintenance tool is ripping us off. Fat vegans become and stay fat by eating junk instead of food... and by not exercising enough, if at all.

A Vergnaud et al. Meat consumption and prospective weight change in participants of the EPIC-PANACEA study. *Am J Clin Nutr.* 2010 Aug;92(2):398-407.

"Total meat consumption was positively associated with weight gain in men and women, in normal-weight and overweight subjects, and in smokers and nonsmokers. With adjustment for estimated energy intake, an increase in meat intake of 250 g/d (e.g., one steak at '450 kcal) would lead to a 2-kg higher weight gain after 5 y (95% CI: 1.5, 2.7 kg). Positive associations were observed for red meat, poultry, and processed meat... Our results suggest that a decrease in meat consumption may improve weight management."

Osteoporosis
P. Appleby, A. Roddam, N. Allen, T. Key. Comparative fracture risk in vegetarians and nonvegetarians in epic-oxford. *Eur J Clin Nutr*, 61(12):1400-1406, 2007.

Here's some contradictory evidence... there are vegans in the UK who're not eating enough leafy greens and other calcium-containing plants, and the result is increased risk of bone fracture:

"The higher fracture rate among vegans in this study appears to reflect their markedly lower mean calcium intake... The percentage of subjects consuming less than 700 mg/day calcium was 15.0 for meat eaters, 15.9 for fish eaters, 18.6 for vegetarians and **76.1 for vegans**." That's an astonishing difference – what are you vegans eating in the UK, for crying out loud? There can't be many Planters among you; and plenty of Junkers. Get a grip, dear Limey vegans – you're making the rest of us look bad.

Also of interest from this paper: "Meat eaters had the highest mean BMI [weighed the most] and tended to be the least active group, with vegans having the lowest mean BMI whilst reporting the highest levels of walking, cycling and vigorous exercise."

K Michaelsson et al. Milk intake and risk of mortality and fractures in women and men: cohort studies. *BMJ*. 2014 Oct 28;349:g6015.

"What this study adds: A high milk intake in both sexes is associated with higher mortality and fracture rates and with higher levels of oxidative stress and inflammatory biomarkers. Such a pattern was not observed with high intake of fermented milk products."

This study confirms the epidemiology of osteoporosis, which shows that the populations who consume the most dairy products have some of the brittlest bones. Keeping in mind that lactose tolerance is a genetic quirk found mainly among people of northern European descent, it's instructive then that the women of the following European nations all suffer high rates of bone disease (>300 per 100,000): The UK, Ireland, Iceland, Norway, Sweden, Denmark, Switzerland, Germany, Czech Republic, Italy, Slovenia, Slovakia, Hungary, Greece and Turkey. The women of Portugal, Spain, France and the Netherlands all have medium rates (>200 per 100,000).

Milk defenders and promoters will say that it's all the sugar these people eat. I agree: it's the milk sugar (and the milk proteins and… and… and…)

There's an interesting map showing this information at http://www.iofbonehealth.org/facts-and-statistics/hip-fracture-incidence-map.

Indians consume mainly fermented milk products, which aren't as bone-destructive as whole milk. Africans have strong bones and consume very little milk. Ditto for China. Sadly, the Chinese living in Taiwan have really taken to dairy products recently – "One local dairy farm imported 1,200 heifers in 2011, which is expected to boost production over the medium term" and "On the import side, the United States overtook New Zealand as the largest supplier of cheese to Taiwan during the first seven months of 2012," according to the USDA'S Foreign Agricultural Service GAIN Report Number TW12032 – and the lactose-intolerant, cheese-eating Taiwanese too have high rates of osteoporosis.

While the lactase mutation may have been beneficial to some of us in prehistory, it's definitely not worth taking advantage of now.

(And I didn't even mention the aging and inflammatory effects of milk's D-galactose.)

Parkinson's "disease"

H. Chen, E. O'Reilly, M. L. McCullough, C. Rodriguez, M. A. Schwarzschild, E. E. Calle, M. J. Thun, and A. Ascherio. Consumption of dairy products and risk of Parkinson's disease. *Am. J. Epidemiol.*, 165(9):998-1006, 2007.

"Diet may play an important role in the etiology of Parkinson's disease, either by altering the oxidative balance in the brain or by serving as a vehicle for environmental neurotoxins... dairy consumption may increase the risk of Parkinson's disease, particularly in men."

Dairy, because of what's in it naturally and because of environmental toxins. Coffee is protective against Parkinson's.

Pre-diabetes

J Tuomilehto et al. Prevention of type 2 diabetes mellitus by changes in lifestyle among subjects with impaired glucose tolerance. *New England Journal of Medicine* 2001 344(18):1343–1350.

"Type 2 diabetes can be prevented by changes in the lifestyles of high-risk subjects... Each subject in the intervention group received individualized counseling aimed at reducing weight, total intake of fat, and intake of saturated fat and increasing intake of fiber and physical activity."

Planting plus exercise stops pre-diabetes progressing to diabetes. Actually, they reverse pre-diabetes, a "disease" in its own right. Here's one of the ways Planting rids us of pre-diabetes:

S Chuengsamarn et al. Curcumin extract for prevention of type 2 diabetes. *Diabetes Care.* 2012 Nov;35(11):2121-7.

"...curcumin extract was able to substantially and significantly prevent T2DM development in the prediabetic population (**0% of curcumin-treated subjects developed DM**, whereas 16.4% of placebo-treated subjects developed DM). In addition, we found that curcumin intervention improved β-cell functions... curcumin treatment may result in better β-cell function in the prediabetic population."

Turmeric and other spices are highly concentrated stores of phytochemicals and have remarkable preventive and healing properties.

Premature puberty

K. Maruyama, T. Oshima, and K. Ohyama. Exposure to exogenous estrogen through intake of commercial milk produced from pregnant cows. *Pediatr Int*, 52(1):33-38, 2010.

"The present data on men and children indicate that estrogens in milk were absorbed, and gonadotropin secretion was suppressed, followed by a decrease in testosterone secretion. Sexual maturation of prepubertal children could be affected by the ordinary intake of cow milk."

Cow's milk is not food for humans; not if it makes 8-year-old girls start growing adult breasts. Ten-year-old minds in 20-year-old bodies is what drives STDs, teenage pregnancies and much of the abortion demand.

It's the milk, stupid, with its huge load of hormones... and the phthalates... and the other endocrine disruptors...

Prostate cancer

Ornish D, Weidner G, Fair WR, Marlin R, Pettengill EB, Raisin CJ, Dunn-Emke S, Crutchfield L, Jacobs FN, Barnard RJ, Aronson WJ, McCormac P, McKnight DJ, Fein JD, Dnistrian AM, Weinstein J, Ngo TH, Mendell NR, Carroll PR. Intensive lifestyle changes may affect the progression of prostate cancer. *J Urol.*, 174(3):1065-9; discussion 1069-70, 2005.

"...intensive changes in diet and lifestyle may beneficially affect the progression of early prostate cancer... Patients with low grade prostate cancer were able to make and maintain comprehensive lifestyle changes for at least 1 year, resulting in significant decreases in serum PSA and a lower likelihood of standard treatment."

Planting has the power to reverse prostate cancer.

Ornish D, Magbanua MJ, Weidner G, Weinberg V, Kemp C, Green C, Mattie MD, Marlin R, Simko J, Shinohara K, Haqq CM, Carroll PR. Changes in prostate gene expression in men undergoing an intensive nutrition and lifestyle intervention. *Proc Natl Acad Sci U S A.* 17;105(24):8369-74, 2008.

"In conclusion, the GEMINAL study suggests that intensive nutrition and lifestyle changes may modulate gene expression in the prostate."

Planting is epigenetically beneficial; Meating never is.

Rheumatoid arthritis

P Tangvoranuntakul et al. Human uptake and incorporation of an immunogenic nonhuman dietary sialic acid. *Proc Natl Acad Sci U S A*. 2003 Oct 14;100(21):12045-50.

"The small amounts of Neu5Gc in normal tissues also raise the possibility that anti-Neu5Gc antibodies are involved in autoimmunity. In this regard, it is interesting that vegetarian diet has been suggested to improve rheumatoid arthritis."

Neu5Gc is an "inflammatory meat molecule" made by the mammals we eat but not by us. Not for two or three million years or so.

J. McDougall et al. Effects of a very low-fat, vegan diet in subjects with rheumatoid arthritis. *J Altern Complement Med*, 8(1):71-75, 2002.

"...patients with moderate-to-severe RA, who switch to a very low-fat, vegan diet can experience significant reductions in RA symptoms."

Planting improves inflammatory conditions such as arthritis; Meating makes them worse.

Sciatica

P Leino-Arjas et al. Serum lipids in relation to sciatica among Finns. *Atherosclerosis*. 2008 Mar;197(1):43-9.

"Atherosclerosis of arteries supplying the lumbar region has been suggested as a mechanism leading to intervertebral disc degeneration and sciatica... Independent of BMI and other possible confounders, clinically assessed sciatica in men was associated with levels of atherogenic serum lipids."

The cholesterol Low-Carb Bullshit Artists tell us not to worry about is what causes sciatica and spinal degeneration... and erectile dysfunction... and...

Sexual dysfunction

K Esposito et al. Hyperlipidemia and sexual function in premenopausal women. *J Sex Med*. 2009 Jun;6(6):1696-703.

"Women with hyperlipidemia [high cholesterol] have significantly lower FSFI-domain scores [Female Sexual Function Index] as compared with age-matched women without hyperlipidemia... women with hyperlipidemia reported **significantly lower arousal, orgasm, lubrication, and satisfaction** scores than control women. Based on the total FSFI score, 51% of women with hyperlipidemia had scores of 26 or less, indicating sexual dysfunction, as compared with 21% of women without hyperlipidemia."

Esposito et al set very high LDL-cholesterol levels, so the chances are the 21% mentioned above also weren't Planters (who are the only people to have optimum animal fat and cholesterol intakes of zero.)

SIDS (Sudden Infant Death Syndrome) ~ Crib Death
J Wasilewska et al. Cow's-milk-induced infant apnoea with increased serum content of bovine β-casomorphin-5. *J Pediatr Gastroenterol Nutr.* 2011 Jun;52(6):772-5.

"We report a case of a breast-fed infant with recurrent apnoea episodes, which have always been preceded by his mother's consumption of fresh cows' milk. A biochemical examination has revealed a high level of β-casomorphin-5 (BCM-5) in the child's serum. We speculate that it is an opioid activity that may have a depressive effect on the respiratory centre of the central nervous system and induce a phenomenon called milk apnoea."

This is how the casomorphin in cows' milk depresses the breathing center in the brains of infants, causing them to die suddenly in their sleep.

Stroke (Cerebrovascular "disease")
JD Spence, DJA Jenkins, J Davignon. Egg yolk consumption and carotid plaque. *Atherosclerosis* 2012 224(2):469–473.

"TPA [total plaque area, a measure of ill-health in the carotid arteries supplying blood to the brain] increases exponentially with smoking pack-years [a measure of cigarette smoking]. TPA increases exponentially with egg-yolk years. The effect size of egg yolks appears to be approximately 2/3 that of smoking. Probably egg yolks should be avoided by persons at risk of vascular disease."

Who's at risk of vascular "disease", putting themselves at risk of stroke? Meaters and Junkers. And Smokers. So, to prevent strokes, who shouldn't eat eggs? People who eat eggs!

Sudden Cardiac Death
Kong MH, Fonarow GC, Peterson ED, Curtis AB, Hernandez AF, Sanders GD, Thomas KL, Hayes DL, Al-Khatib SM. Systematic review of the incidence of sudden cardiac death in the United States. *J Am Coll Cardiol.* 2011 Feb 15;57(7):794-801.

"In the United States, cardiovascular disease was the underlying cause of one of every 2.9 deaths occurring in 2006. The proportion of these deaths that is sudden has been estimated to be as high as 50%, making sudden cardiac death (SCD) the most common cause of death in this country."

One of several reasons why Meaters and Junkers are more prone to SCD is because of a deficiency in magnesium, the metal at the heart of the chlorophyll molecule. Understandably, as chlorophyll is the green pigment in plants, Planters aren't deficient in magnesium.

M Guasch-Ferre et al, PREDIMED Study Group. Dietary Magnesium Intake Is Inversely Associated with Mortality in Adults at High Cardiovascular Disease Risk 1. *J Nutr.* 2014 Jan;144(1):55-60.

"Dietary magnesium intake was inversely associated with mortality risk in Mediterranean individuals at high risk of CVD [cardiovascular disease].

Ulcerative colitis

A Birkett, J Muir, J Phillips, G Jones, K O'Dea. Resistant starch lowers fecal concentrations of ammonia and phenols in humans. *Am J Clin Nutr.* 1996 May;63(5):766-72.

"During the high-RS [resistant starch] diet daily excretion of fecal nitrogen increased... and excretion of fecal phenols fell ... Fecal concentrations of ammonia decreased... and phenols decreased... pH decreased from 6.4... to 6.2... during the high-RS period. These results suggest that RS significantly attenuates the accumulation of potentially harmful byproducts of protein fermentation in the human colon."

For colon health, Meating bad, Planting good.

SU Christi et al. Antagonistic effects of sulfide and butyrate on proliferation of colonic mucosa: a potential role for these agents in the pathogenesis of ulcerative colitis. *Dig Dis Sci.* 1996 Dec;41(12):2477-81.

"...feces of patients with ulcerative colitis uniformly contain sulfate reducing bacteria. Sulfide produced by these bacteria... may be involved in the pathogenesis of ulcerative colitis... Our data support a possible role of sulfide in the pathogenesis of UC and confirm the role of butyrate in the regulation of colonic proliferation and in the treatment of UC."

Again, Planting feeds our gut bacteria and they produce beneficial butyrate, while Meating produces pathogenic hydrogen sulfide.

Urinary tract infections (UTIs)

L. Jakobsen et al. Is Escherichia coli urinary tract infection a zoonosis? Proof of direct link with production animals and meat. *Eur. J. Clin. Microbiol. Infect. Dis.* 2012 31(6):1121 – 1129.

"This study showed a clonal link between E. coli from meat and humans, providing solid evidence that UTI is zoonosis [animal-borne disease]."

Bacteria from animals, particularly chickens, cause urinary tract infections in ten million American Meater women each year.

Bacterial vaginosis

N. Ahluwalia, H. Grandjean. Nutrition, an under-recognized factor in bacterial vaginosis. *J. Nutr.* 2007 137(9):1997 - 1998

"…lower serum concentrations of vitamins A, C, and E, and b-carotene were associated with BV, and lower iron status… was associated with increased prevalence of Candida colonization."

The more nutrient-dense our diet is, and the higher the pH of our vaginas remains, the less we'll suffer from bacterial infections of the vagina. In other words… the more Planter our diet is, the healthier our vaginas.

Being high in saturated fats, both Junking (cakes and cookies) and Meating (dairy and chickens) tend to raise vaginal pH and encourage unhealthy bacteria to blossom.

Yeast infections ~ *Candida*

LA David et al. Diet rapidly and reproducibly alters the human gut microbiome. *Nature* 505, 559–563 (23 January 2014).

"Significant increases in *Penicillium*-related fungi were observed, along with significant decreases in the concentration of *Debaryomyces* and a *Candida* sp."

Part of the reason why Planters get fewer yeast infections is that our gut bacteria are unfriendly to pathogenic species of yeasts and friendly to beneficial species. *Candida albicans* et al can only flourish and 'bloom' in conditions made propitious for them by Meating or Junking.

~

References to papers on animal deficiencies

MH Carlsen et al. The total antioxidant content of more than 3100 foods, beverages, spices, herbs and supplements used worldwide. *Nutr J*. 2010 Jan 22;9:3.

"…there are several thousand-fold differences in antioxidant content of foods. Spices, herbs and supplements include the most antioxidant rich products in our study, some exceptionally high. Berries, fruits, nuts, chocolate, vegetables and products thereof constitute common foods and beverages with high antioxidant values.

This database is to our best knowledge the most comprehensive Antioxidant Food Database published and it shows that **plant-based foods introduce significantly more antioxidants into human diet than non-plant foods** [animals]."

Also, it's important to "understand the role of dietary phytochemical antioxidants in the prevention of cancer, cardiovascular diseases, diabetes and other **chronic diseases related to oxidative stress**."

The animals we eat **cause oxidative stress** and are pathetically deficient in antioxidants. Some plants contain more than one hundred thousand times as many antioxidants as animals do; but to be fair, on average, the common food plants we eat most often contain about 64 times more antioxidants than their animal counterparts.

Animals are poor food substitutes and should be treated as emergency rations only.

Nishi K, Kondo A, Okamoto T, Nakano H, Daifuku M, Nishimoto S, Ochi K, Takaoka T, Sugahara T. Immunostimulatory in vitro and in vivo effects of a water-soluble extract from kale. *Biosci Biotechnol Biochem*. 2011;75(1):40-6.

"Since IgA [immunoglobulin A, an antibody produced by plasma, or white blood cells] is the predominant Ig in normal intestinal mucosa, accounting for 70-90% of all Igs in GALT [gut-associated lymphoid tissue, the gastrointestinal tract's immune system] and thus plays a pivotal role in host defense, the intake of kale might provide a beneficial effect on humans to enhance the defense against such pathogens as viruses, bacteria and toxins [all of which come overwhelmingly from animals]. The immune-stimulating effect will provide an additional advantage of kale, as well as its antioxidative capacity and other effects."

Animals provide the antigens, or foreign attackers; plants provide the antibodies, or local defense force. So which is food?

Chen T, Yan F, Qian J, Guo M, Zhang H, Tang X, Chen F, Stoner GD, Wang X. Randomized phase II trial of lyophilized strawberries in patients with dysplastic precancerous lesions of the esophagus. *Cancer Prev Res* (Phila). 2012 Jan;5(1):41-50.

Strawberries are protective against esophageal cancer. Not this or that or the other extracted, refined chemical from strawberries: whole strawberries.

Animals cause cancers; plants heal them.

SS Percival et al. Bioavailability of Herbs and Spices in Humans as Determined by ex vivo Inflammatory Suppression and DNA Strand Breaks. *J Am Coll Nutr.* 2012 31(4):288-294.

Don't get put off by the technical language; just take in the fact that the named herbs and spices protect us against DNA damage and cancer:

"Herbs and spices that protected PBMCs against DNA strand breaks were **paprika**, **rosemary**, **ginger**, heat-treated **turmeric**, **sage**, and **cumin**. **Paprika** also appeared to protect cells from normal apoptotic processes... **Clove**, **ginger**, **rosemary**, and **turmeric** were able to significantly reduce oxidized LDL-induced expression of TNF-α.

Serum from those consuming **ginger** reduced all three inflammatory biomarkers. **Ginger**, **rosemary**, and **turmeric** showed protective capacity by both oxidative protection and inflammation measures."

Plants are anti-oxidant, anti-inflammatory and DNA-protective; animals are oxidizing, inflammatory and DNA-disruptive.

Bailey SJ, Winyard P, Vanhatalo A, Blackwell JR, Dimenna FJ, Wilkerson DP, Tarr J, Benjamin N, Jones AM. Dietary nitrate supplementation reduces the O_2 cost of low-intensity exercise and enhances tolerance to high-intensity exercise in humans. *J Appl Physiol.* 2009 Oct;107(4):1144-55.

Now this would seem to be a very important nutrition and sports physiology paper, but I've never seen or heard it mentioned by a single Low-Carb Bullshit Artist, even the world-famous sports physiologists among them.

It appears that beets, beet greens, arugula and other high-nitrate plants can boost our arterial production of NO (nitric oxide) and cause our arteries to dilate to such an extent and supply our muscle cells with so much oxygen that we can do remarkable athletic feats, previously thought to be impossible. For one, we can perform the same amount of work while using less oxygen. For another, we can significantly extend our time to exhaustion while doped up with leafy greens.

Endurance athletes should be greening up as well as carbo-loading. As Michael Greger puts it: "Beets [have been] found to significantly improve athletic performance while reducing oxygen needs, upsetting a fundamental tenet of sports physiology." It's a wee bit technical, but I urge anyone interested in peak performance to read this paper.

Bailey et al say: "It should be stressed that the remarkable reduction in the O_2 cost of submaximal cycle exercise following dietary supplementation with inorganic nitrate in the form of a natural food product cannot be achieved by any other known means, including long-term endurance exercise training."

I'll translate into English from Bailey's low-key science-speak: "This is freaking amazing! We thought this was impossible… rewrite all the sports physiology books."

Animals don't do this, because they're not food. Only whole plants truly nourish human beings.

And that's me done with providing references to great 'microscopic' science. It's time now to break out our endoscopes… our gastroscopes and enteroscopes, depending on which end we're going to scope, front or rear, top or bottom.

~

All together now...

Now that we've gotten all the reductionist science out of the way, let's look at the big picture of nutrition.

We don't eat single 'nutrients'; we eat foods or non-foods; plants or animals and junk, and they contain different groups of nutrients and non-nutrients.

Studying each dietary 'ingredient' individually, in a reductionist manner, is obviously helpful, but we need to see how they all work together if we're to understand how the human organism works as a gestalt.

We don't eat saturated or trans fats or cholesterol on their own. The animals that contain these non-nutrients also harbor cadaverine, putrescine, alpha-gal, amyloid, arachidonic acid, estrogens, harmane, purines, sulfur-containing amino acids and dozens of the other malefic Meater components which we met in Part 1; plus some of the dozens of pathogenic germs and worms we met in Part 2, plus a whole slew of the environmental poisons we met in Part 3. And they all collaborate to harm us, their total carnage being way worse than the sum of their toxic parts.

Imagine for a moment that we're in an auto workshop. A mechanic is working there on a PVT, a 'post-vintage thoroughbred,' a beaut of a car not old enough to be called vintage. [Like me.] She's taken all the pieces apart, and laid them lovingly out on a giant tarp, ready to check and refurbish and oil them, before she puts the whole thing back together again. It looks like a real-life exploded diagram, only without the labels.

Okay, that's what I've done so far with animals and, to a lesser extent, junk. I've laid out all the parts, like the TMAO, the heme iron, the heterocyclic amines – they're all lying there, waiting for me to reassemble them.

All that's passed has been prolog to this moment, in which I try to emulate Prof. T. Colin Campbell's *Whole* approach to nutrition. Keeping in mind that the processes I'm about to describe take place together or shortly after each other, and that some of the processes can build up over decades of Meater mal-nutrition, let's see what happens when we put pieces of animal in our mouths and swallow them.

Here goes...

Down the hatch...

A Turd's Eye View of an Animal Meal

Meating's effects on ingestion, digestion, metabolism and excretion

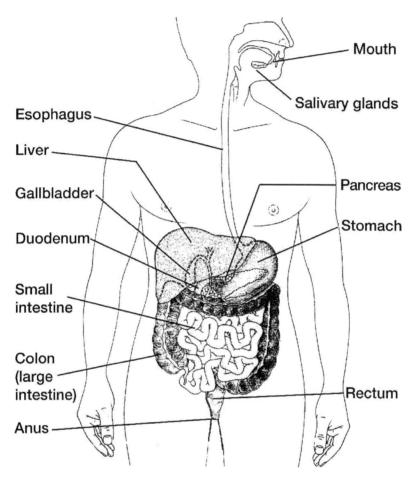

Alimentary, my dear Watson (Source unknown – my apologies – please let me
know if it's yours and I'll remedy the situation.)

The Mouth

If we recall from the opening paragraph of Michael Moss's *Salt Sugar Fat*,
"Our bodies are hard-wired for sweets." Our mouths are all about sugar.
Carbohydrate digestion begins immediately. There are barely any sugars in
animals besides some glycogen in their muscles and lactose, so only milk-

fed human babies begin digesting energy-rich animal sugars straight away. In adults, sugars come from whole plants, or should.

There are three types of salivary glands in the mouth: the sublingual (below the tongue), the submandibular (below the lower jaw bone, or mandible) and the parotid, the largest ones in our cheeks. Their watery secretions contain the carb-cracking enzyme salivary amylase, a.k.a. ptyalin.

Our teeth – of which we have two matching plates of 16, top and bottom – are outstanding slicers and grinders of fibrous plants, with their tough cellulose cell walls. They're not very well adapted to tearing and chewing animals, the cells of which have outer membranes rather than walls.

The shape and size and spacing of our teeth, and our jaw musculature and hinging, allowing for side-to-side motion, also reflect our essential Planter nature.

On page 5 of his "The Comparative Anatomy of Eating," Dr. Milton Mills says:

> "Human teeth are also similar to those found in other herbivores with the exception of the canines (the canines of some of the apes are elongated and are thought to be used for display and/or defense). Our teeth are rather large and usually abut against one another. The incisors are flat and spade-like, useful for peeling, snipping and biting relatively soft materials. The canines are neither serrated nor conical, but are flattened, blunt and small and function like incisors. The premolars and molars are squarish, flattened and nodular, and used for crushing, grinding and pulping non-coarse foods."

> Human saliva contains the carbohydrate-digesting enzyme, salivary amylase. This enzyme is responsible for the majority of starch digestion."

On page 2, Dr. Mills says:

> "The saliva of carnivorous animals does not contain digestive enzymes. When eating, a mammalian carnivore gorges itself rapidly and does not chew its food. Since proteolytic (protein-digesting) enzymes cannot be liberated in the mouth due to the danger of autodigestion (damaging the oral cavity), carnivores do not need to mix their food with saliva; they simply bite off huge chunks of meat and swallow them whole."

We don't have to travel very far through the digestive tract to realize that – based on our physiology and anatomy – we're not Meaters. Just because we practice omnivorism doesn't make us functional omnivores.

(That some Meaters claim we're supposed to eat animals because we have teeth called canines is hilarious. Our canines are sometimes called 'eye teeth.' Does that mean I'll be able to see in the dark if I walk around with my mouth open?)

Nevertheless (after we've stabbed the beast with our steely knives instead of using our teeth for the initial slicing), our jaws and teeth are versatile enough to allow us to break down animals mechanically into swallowable pieces. And then our saliva coats them and makes them easier to swallow.

Before that happens, the introduction of unfriendly bacteria can disturb the beneficial bacteria that live around our tongues, which are responsible for nitrate metabolism and NO production, so important for arterial dilation.

A mouthful of animal alerts our immune system to the presence of antigens (foreign invaders) and may start producing antibodies. Aphthous ulcers, or canker sores are, most often, an immune response to dairy products.

When it's time to swallow, our tongues and cheeks and palates all get in on the action, and the mouthful moves past the epiglottis, through the pharynx (preferably not into the larynx, or wind pipe in front of it) and into…

The Esophagus
The esophagus is a muscular, pink 18-inch-long tube that connects our throats to our stomachs. Proving that we come from outer space, our esophagi can propel food upward against gravity, when we're upside down, by muscular contractions similar to peristalsis in our intestines. (Kidding.) Its narrow diameter is best adapted to passing well-chewed fibrous plants, not large chunks of flesh. 99.9999% of the time, or so, Meaters survive the swallowing process. Occasionally we choke to death on a gobbet of flesh, if un-Heimliched, or we get punctured by a bone.

The esophagus passes through our chest cavities, in between the lungs, then behind our hearts and through the sheet of muscle that controls our breathing – the diaphragm – and so into our stomachs, in our abdomens. The hole in the diaphragm through with the esophagus passes is called the esophageal hiatus. At the bottom of the esophagus is a ring of muscles that closes up to prevent acid from the stomach refluxing into the esophagus.

We'll come back to hiatus hernia and gastro-esophageal reflux disease later.

The Stomach

When a bolus, or ball of anything we eat hits our stomach after transiting the esophagus, protein digestion begins. Our stomach linings are amazing. They're made out of proteins and yet they're able to secrete hydrochloric acid and a stew of protein-cracking enzymes – pepsin, trypsin and chymotrypsin – without auto-digesting themselves.

They do this in a most cunning way. There are mucus-secreting cells that provide a barrier against the food/acid/enzyme mix and, also, the acid is secreted in such a way that it only becomes activated in the lumen, or chamber, of the stomach. Amazing.

Protein breakdown happens in three ways – via acid and enzymes, and also by the churning action of the stomach. It's a muscular pouch and its internal surface has folds, or rugae, which act in the same way as the turbulence-creating vertical fins in blenders to mix things up well.

While quite acidic, our gastric juices are nowhere as low in pH (more acidic) as those of omnivores or carnivores. Even so, the higher protein load of animals is problematic, in that it requires a more acidic environment and a longer time to break down the peptide chains of amino acids. Meaters are more prone to ulceration. (Aspirin-taking Meaters are much more prone to ulcers than Planters, who get their salicylic acid from plants.)

Animals stay in our stomachs for longer than plants, because Meaters are getting up to triple the amount of proteins than Planters do, and both groups in the US are eating more than is necessary. "Getting our protein" is a persistent myth. It would take great skill to plan a diet that didn't provide enough proteins if we're eating enough calories.

Going back to the esophagus. Over time, a constant assault of animals and junk such as hot beverages, alcohol, phosphoric acid-containing sodas and overly hot (as in spicy) foods can damage the relatively weak muscles of the lower esophageal sphincter (LES), allowing stomach acid to reflux into the esophagus, especially when we lie down.

Unlike the stomach, the esophagus has no mucous barrier to acid, and the acid can burn the inner lining of cells and cause bleeding, a condition called esophagitis, and, if it continues, cause a long-term inflammatory condition known as GERD, or gastro-esophageal reflux disease, which in turn can become chronic Barrett's esophagus or even lethal esophageal cancer.

Fortunately, we can minimize the dangers of these conditions. The main reason we create stomach acid is to deal with proteins. Firstly, animals contain more than plants. Secondly, we eat way more animals than we need. So, if we're Planting we get about half the proteins that Meaters consume (and that's probably still more than we need). That's helpful when we're faced with GERD or cancer.

In his terrific video, *Digestion Made Easy – A Journey Through Your Amazing Digestive System*, Michael Klaper, MD, suggests we do the following to combat GERD:

- raise the head of our beds 4 to 6 inches to prevent reflux at night;
- eat high-protein meals early in the day; high-carb in the evenings;
- try "herbal considerations" such as slippery elm, deglycyrrhizinated licorice (DGL) and cabbage juice;
- get a test done for *Helicobacter pylori*, an ulcer-causing bacterium;
- as a last resort, use acid-blocking drugs for the six weeks or so it takes our esophagi to rejuvenate.

The other problem I alluded to before – hiatus or hiatal hernia – is one of the pressure "diseases" we encountered earlier when we discussed constipation. Constipation (which is common among Meaters and Junkers) or being obese (not a Planter condition) can create sufficient pressure to force a part of our stomach or esophagus (which are supposed to stay below our diaphragms in our abdomens) up through the esophageal hiatus – the gap in the diaphragm through which the esophagus passes – and into our chest cavities or thoraxes. The LES, or lower esophageal sphincter then loses all function and reflux occurs as a matter of course, and most every time we lie down.

Meating + Junking → constipation + obesity → hiatus hernia → esophagitis → GERD → esophageal cancer.

We need to snap this chain, as early as possible. To me that doesn't mean taking fiber supplements or going on a weight-loss diet; it means stopping Meating and Junking.

Our meal is now ready to leave the stomach. The animal parts we're following have had their proteins cracked into smaller peptide units, made up of shorter strings of amino acids. Nothing much has happened to fats other than being churned into smaller droplets: no chemical breakdown yet.

(Carbohydrate digestion, which starts in the vaguely alkaline mouth, lies dormant in the highly acidic stomach, as the amylase enzyme is diluted and deactivated.)

The next stop on the digestion train is the small intestine, specifically the C-shaped first 12 inches called the duodenum (the Greek for 12 inches being 'duodeni.') The last station in the stomach is the very strong muscular sphincter at the bottom end of the stomach, the pyloric sphincter. But there's a problem.

The Duodenum

Form follows function… and the function of the duodenum is to continue cracking carbs and proteins, while starting to crack fats. It works best at an alkaline pH. Because of its function, the duodenum's form lacks mucus-secreting cells, so how are we going to keep it safe from the acid we're about to inject?

Ladies and gentlemen, I give you…

The Pancreas

Liver, Gallbladder, Pancreas and Bile Passage

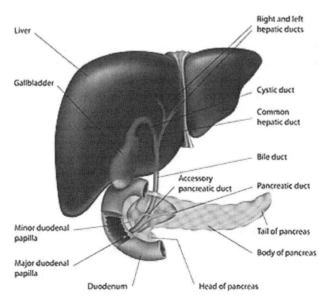

Liver, gallbladder et al. http://images.medicinenet.com/images/appictures/liver-disease-s2-what-is-liver-disease.jpg

The pancreas is a glandular organ that nestles within the curve of the duodenum, behind the stomach

When the stomach's work is done, the pyloric sphincter opens briefly and it jets through a tablespoon or two of chyme, a gruel of semi-digested, acidified nutrients, into the duodenum.

At the same time, our new friend, the pancreas, secretes a dose of digestive enzymes into the duodenum, along with a spritz of bicarbonate, which has a pH of 8.8. When chyme meets pancreatic juices, pancreatic juices win and neutralize the acid, and the pH of the duodenum settles down to about 8.0, which is the perfect alkalinity for carbohydrate digestion to continue. (7 is neutral.)

The glands that make up the pancreas come in two varieties: endocrine (which secrete their hormones directly into the bloodstream) and exocrine (which secrete their enzymes into ducts). The digestive enzymes come from the pancreas's alpha- or exocrine glands; two hormones – insulin and glucagon – come from the beta- or endocrine cells in the islets of Langerhans within the pancreas.) We'll have a lot more to say later about insulin and it's less famous reciprocal, glucagon.

The pancreas secretes about 8 cups of juice a day. The digestive enzymes in it are

- Amylase, which continues the breakdown of carbohydrates (starch) into simple sugars, begun by salivary amylase;
- Proteases, which break proteins and peptides into amino acids. They also help combat parasites such as yeast, bacteria and protozoa (which are made out of proteins); and
- Lipase, which helps break down fats.

That's the order in which digestion proceeds – carbs first, then proteins, then fats – and that should give us some idea about their relative physiological importance: carbs to power us; proteins for making enzymes and (a little) for meat-making; and fats for future energy storage, and other jobs like maintaining cell membranes and nerve sheaths.

So, in the duodenum, starch and protein digestion continue, and fat digestion begins. Again, fats are more complicated than starch and protein.

Our intestines and bloodstreams are watery, or aqueous environments, and oil and water don't mix. So we need a detergent to emulsify the fats to make them water-soluble. Enter…

The Liver and Gallbladder

The liver is our "master chemist": it takes in all the nutrients we eat and digest and take up in our blood, and from them it creates thousands of different useful compounds. (There is a porous membrane which allows just-about-everything to enter the liver – this makes it susceptible to damage by toxins such as industrial pollutants and alcohol.)

One hepatic compound we're interested in for digestion is a yellowish fluid called bile, or gall. The liver takes cholesterol and makes bile out of it.

When some chyme enters the duodenum, our pancreases release alkaline pancreatic juices full of enzymes. The lipase starts fat breakdown, releasing smaller fat droplets.

At the same time, the liver releases bile into its duct system, it flows down (past a turnoff to the gallbladder, the between-meal storage depot for bile) and enters the duodenum at the sphincter of Oddi. Bile is electrically charged, with positive and negative ends. The negative ends attach to fat droplets, leaving the positive ends to interact with water (consisting of H^+ and O^- ions.) The fats are now soluble in the water and can be absorbed into the bloodstream and transported to the liver.

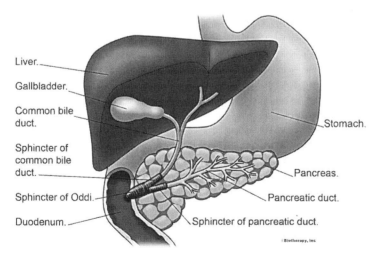

The Sphincter of Oddi, at the end of the common bile duct and the pancreatic duct
- irishdysautonomia.wordpress.com

703

When we've finished processing the entire meal, bile continues to collect in the bile duct system above the sphincter of Oddi. When it meets the turnoff to the gallbladder, instead of backing up into the liver, it heads up the side duct and gets stored in the gallbladder. At the onset of digestion of the next meal, the gallbladder squeezes a spritz of bile back down the duct and into the duodenum.

Gallstones

Meating and Junking cause problems in the biliary system by providing excess cholesterol. When we eat animal and junk fats (saturated and trans fats, and hydrogenated oils) we stimulate the liver to produce excess cholesterol. There's only so much cholesterol that bile salts can hold in solution and, when the bile is saturated, cholesterol crystallizes out and forms gallstones. Besides being excruciating – imagine the feeling when the gallbladder contracts and tries to shove large crystalline stones down a narrow pipe – the stones get covered with intestinal bacteria, causing inflammation and infection. Over time, the gallbladder lining is destroyed and loses all function. Every year >700,000 American Meaters and Junkers have their gallbladders surgically removed.

Gallstones aren't the only problem though…

Animals and junk contain no fiber. Fiber is the indigestible-by-humans-but-digestible-by-healthy-gut-bacteria starch found in whole plants. Not only does it have valuable, unique nutrients bound to it; not only does it bulk out our stools and make them easy to pass; fiber acts as a brush that sweeps through our intestines, binding up excess cholesterol and heavy metals and other nasties, and otherwise keeping our guts (and us) healthy.

Fiber performs a host of important functions:

- Because whole plants are low in energy and high in bulk, our stomachs fill up sooner, giving us a sense of fullness or satiety
- It bulks out our stools, making them activate the pressure receptors in our bowels, telling peristaltic waves to move our garbage along
- It holds more moisture, making our stools softer and easier to evacuate
- It binds up heavy metals, excess cholesterol and carcinogenic bile acids
- It removes excess carcinogenic estrogens from our system

- It creates a health gut flora, which keeps pathogenic strains of microbes in check, preventing intestinal and extra-intestinal infections; the ones which kill tens of thousands of Meaters annually, and
- It feeds our gut flora, which in turn produce cancer-fighting substance such as butyrate and lignans.

High fiber diets and healthy intestines are synonymous. Meating and Junking are potentially lethal fiber-deficiency diseases.

What we eat affects our

Transit time

When we're Planters, a meal takes 24 hours to enter our mouths, be digested and absorbed, and for our fecal waste to exit our poop chutes. Meaters and Junkers can take a week or more to expel a meal. That's asking for trouble: days of extra, unnecessary exposure to carcinogens, parasites and toxins. Constipation helps cause cancer.

We're not just what we eat. And we're not just what we absorb. We are what we don't excrete. When we're constipated, we don't excrete a whole lot… which you can read either way you like.

Meating creates constipation. Anyone who isn't having at least one excellent bowel movement a day is ill. To have only a single bowel movement a week, as happens to many Meaters, isn't only to be full of shit; it's to court dis-ass-ster [dis-arse-ster in the UK]. Sorry, it's not a laughing matter.

If we're constipated, we know we're malnourished, and mal-nutrition is what causes heart "disease", stroke, cancer, hypertension, and the endless roll call of "diseases" of Western civilization. We're eating ourselves to death, and constipation is a fire alarm that should cause us to exit the building; instead, to our peril, we switch off the smoke detector with drugs or supplements and ignore it.

Our health is in our own hands. We can either eat whole plants, especially water- and fiber-rich fruit, and not cause constipation or cancer, or we can buy supplements from the Atkins or paleo punters to try and reverse the constipating and cancer-causing conditions their dietstyles cause.

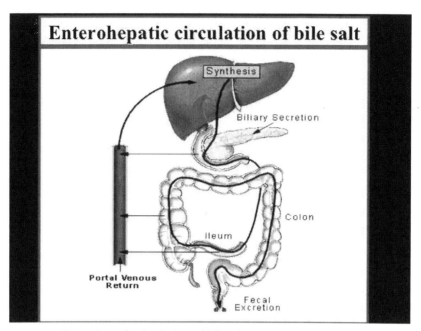

Enterohepatic circulation of bile salt. Image: slideshare.net

Our bodies are conservative, in more ways than one. They don't do radical. And they conserve the nutrients and metabolites they need. Why excrete stuff if you can use it again?

The enterohepatic circulation of bile

Enterohepatic means 'gut – liver.' Most of our bile gets recycled. Before the end of the small intestine, which we're about to get up close to, the bile passes through the gut wall along with absorbed nutrients and gets collected in larger and larger veins until the portal vein enters the liver, where it then fans out and floods our liver cells with nutrients. Our hepatocytes (liver cells) extract the bile and send it back into the duct system for reuse. Excess bile gets discharged into the fecal stream in the large intestine and gets pooped out. Which is good because excess causes cancer. Meaters and Junkers have far more in their feces, and it spends more time there. Hence, their increased risk of colorectal and other cancers.

Breast and prostate cancer

As we saw earlier, women who have few bowel movements are at much greater risk of developing breast cancer. Excess carcinogenic bile acids and carcinogenic cholesterol and carcinogenic estrogens don't get swept out of us when we're fiber-deficient Meaters and Junkers; they re-enter our blood

706

and become hyper-concentrated in breast and prostate tissue at 100x the external level. When we're Planters we have lots of fiber in our guts, which flush out these noxious chemicals. Breast cancer is largely an eating disorder.

Not only does everything happen at once; all parts of us are connected to all the other parts of us – our blood flows everywhere – and what happens in our bowels affects all our body systems. Moving on...

The Small Intestine

The small intestine is the miraculous place where macro-nutrient absorption takes place. By now we've broken down our proteins, starch and fats into their basic units. The small intestine is where these units pass through the gut wall and enter the blood, and make their way to the liver for metabolism.

The small intestine, of which the duodenum is the first foot, is 22 to 30 feet long (or 7 to 9 meters) and its inner lining consists of bajillions of sea anemone-like projections called villi that increase its absorptive area by orders of magnitude. According to Michael Klaper, we each have 'half an NFL football field' of absorptive area in our small intestines.

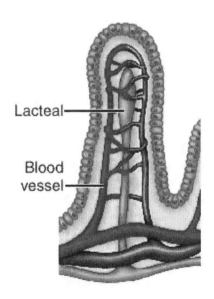

A villus. http://medical-dictionary.thefreedictionary.com/villus

Sugars and amino acids pass through the villi walls and get taken up in the venous return system and make their way to the liver. Fats definitely suffer from the fear of being ordinary: their absorption is different to starch and protein. Instead of entering the veins in the villi, they enter lacteals.

A lacteal is a lymphatic vessel that conveys chyle. And chyle, according to Dorland's Medical Dictionary is "the milky fluid taken up by the lacteals from food in the intestine, consisting of an emulsion of lymph and triglyceride fat (chylomicrons); it passes into the veins by the thoracic duct and mixes with blood," and then makes its way to the liver. There's always one…

The mesenteric system, or the hepatic portal system

As nutrients get absorbed into the villi's veins and lacteals, the blood flows into ever-larger mesenteric veins, which eventually join in our guts' Amazon river, the hepatic portal vein – the doorway to the liver.

By the time we reach the end of the narrow, long small intestine, all of the macronutrients have been absorbed, and most of the bile acids have been reabsorbed.

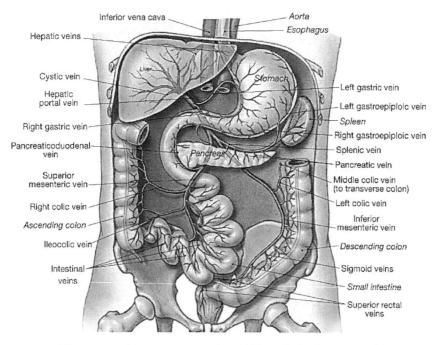

The mesenteric venous system: http://droualb.faculty.mjc.edu/

The terminal end of the small intestine – the ileum – meets the much wider, shorter larger large intestine, or colon, at the ileocecal junction. The first part of the large intestine is called the cecum.

In Planters, about 6 hours have gone by. Meaters and Junkers, with more fats and proteins to process, take hours longer.

PCRM describes the consequences of a high-fat meal very well. High-fat meals are usually Meater- and Junker-catered... Planters should be wary of vegetable oils – they're 100% fat.

The Good Stuff? Think Again...

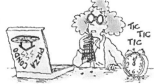

What Happens after Only One High-Fat Meal?

So you've just finished your high fat dinner of a hamburger, cheese pizza or chicken...
What's next?

Immediately...
- Your triglyceride levels, a measurement of fat in your bloodstream, are rising.
- Your cholesterol levels are increasing, contributing to plaque formation.
- Clotting factors in your blood have been activated.

Two hours later...
- Your triglycerides have increased by 60 percent.
- Your blood flow has decreased by half.

Three hours later...
- The lining of your arteries has lost elasticity impeding blood flow.
- Blood vessel function has become abnormal.

Four hours later...
- Your blood has gotten thicker, flowing even slower than it was 2 hours ago.

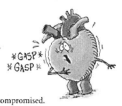

Five hours later...
- Your triglyceride levels have now increased by 150 percent.

Six hours later...
- The anti-inflammatory effect of "good" cholesterol has been significantly compromised.

Consumption of high-fat foods over days, weeks, months, years...
- Saturated fat in your diet has promoted the continuous buildup of plaque in your arteries, reducing blood flow even further.
- Decreased blood flow leads to decreased oxygen supply, which can lead to a heart attack.
- You are in danger of developing fatty liver disease.

Larsen LF, Bladbjerg EM, Jespersen J, Marckmann P. Effects of dietary fat quality and quantity on postprandial activation of blood coagulation factor VII. *Arterioscler Thromb Vasc Biol.* 1997;17:2904-2909.

Vogel RA, Corretti MC, Plotnick GD. Effect of a single high-fat meal on endothelial function in healthy subjects. *Am J Cardiol.* 1997; 79:350-354.

Nicholls SJ, Lundman P, Harmer J, et al. Consumption of saturated fat impairs the anti-inflammatory properties of high-density lipoproteins and endothelial function. *J Am Coll Cardiol.* 2006; 48: 715-720.

Hozumi T, Eisenberg M, Sugioka K, et al. Change in coronary flow reserve on transthoracic Doppler echocardiography after a single high-fat meal in young healthy men. *Ann Intern Med.* 2002;136:523-528.

Post-prandial lipemia.
Source: PCRM (Physicians Committee for Responsible Medicine.)

Now's a good time to talk about

Insulin resistance – pre-diabetes - diabetes

Besides producing digestive juices in its exocrine glands, the pancreas produces two hormones in its endocrine glands, which it secretes directly into our blood.

When glucose appears in our blood, it's the role of hormone #1, insulin, to deliver glucose to individual cells. Insulin uses a key to open a door in our cell membranes, it takes glucose through the door, and then, inside the city, it takes glucose to the cell's power plants, organelles called mitochondria. In the presence of oxygen, glucose gets burned up and produces energy molecules called ATP.

It's insulin's job to deal with glucose when it arrives. It lowers our blood sugar level.

Hormone #2 – glucagon – is the anti-matter to insulin's matter. It raises our blood sugar level when it falls too low. It does this by mobilizing sugar from glycogen, the small short-term sugar store in our muscles.

Insulin and glucagon work together to keep our blood sugar levels within a narrow healthy band.

Normally, glucose comes packaged with fiber and other phytonutrients, and it takes time to break down the starches. Normally, there's a slow, extended release of glucose over many hours. Junking – eating fiber-depleted plants – presents our bodies with an immediate blast of pre-digested glucose. Our blood sugar level spikes up – bang – causing our insulin level to spike up to remove the sugar from our blood – bang – then our blood sugars plummet again – bang – often dropping back below where we started, leaving us exhausted.

It's like teenage sex… wham, bam, thank you, ma'am, over in a flash, then you lie around, depleted, not knowing where to look or what to say.

Over the course of years, we may need to produce more insulin to get the same result. Sugar's just like any drug, that way. By constantly assaulting our pancreases with sugar, we may become resistant to insulin, and set ourselves up for diabetes.

But… that's only the Junker part of the story. Here's the Meater part.

It's not just sugar that causes us to release insulin. Because of the animal fats they contain, which insulin is responsible for ferrying into fat cells, and because of the amino acids they contain, which insulin moves into other body cells for growth and repair, the animals we eat cause an insulin spike similar to that caused by high-glycemic, processed carbs like white sugar. Even though they don't contain any carbs. Insulin isn't only about glucose. Try to find that tidbit in a Low-Carb Bullshit Artist's nutrition comic book.

Then, animal and junk fats cause insulin resistance. Fats block insulin's ability to ferry glucose into our muscle cells, and block insulin from ferrying glucose to our mitochondria inside our cells, causing our pancreases to increase insulin secretion and leading, long-term, to reduced sensitivity and type II diabetes. Nasty sequelae of diabetes – a Meater and Junker affliction – include arterial damage, heart "disease", blindness (diabetic retinopathy), kidney failure, amputations because of gangrene, and dementia.

And while the animal proteins may be damaging and lowering the effectiveness of our pancreatic insulin-making cells (even in cases where type 1 diabetes doesn't arise), the animal fats are sludging up our blood, coating our blood cells and making peripheral circulation difficult, gradually allowing the build-up of crut where it doesn't belong, damaging our eyes with drusen, and other delicate organs with lactic acid and other metabolites.

Insulin resistance is about 'meat + sweet.' It's about the two non-foods: animals *and* junk. Even if we avoid eating animals, we've still got to avoid Junking. Eating high-glycemic, highly processed, industrialized starches and sugars is a sure-fire recipe for IR, diabesity and diabetes.

For Meaters to blame diabetes entirely on 'carbs' is outright wrong. (Planters, the people who eat the highest whole-carb diets have the least obesity, diabetes, heart "disease", stroke, cancer and... you name it.) Still, it's possible for high-animal eaters to be healthy-looking in the short term, when they cut out Junking. Paleo dieters are essentially Planter/Meater hybrids, and they're healthy to the extent that they've cut out Junking, and to the extent that their Planting temporarily masks the ill-effects of Meating.

The process of diabetes can takes place over years and decades, so we're fooled into thinking we're healthy and strong until middle age arrives and, all of a sudden, things start going wrong. Not always decades though: kids now get 'adult onset' diabetes – it's the animals AND it's the junk, and it's the lack of vitamin X - exercise.

We shouldn't let the Low-Carb Bullshit Artists bullshit us that whole carbs cause diabetes. They don't.

Whole carbs are the only food.

Next stop…

The Large Intestine

The large intestine is described as having 5 parts:

- Ascending colon
- Transverse colon
- Descending colon
- Sigmoid colon [S-shaped]
- Rectum [Straight]

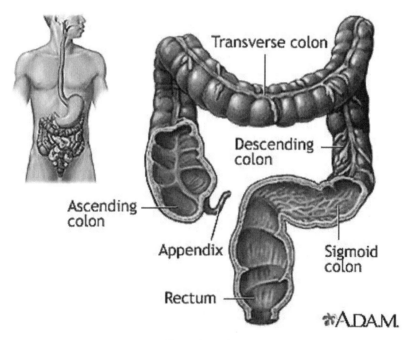

Large intestine:
MedlinePlus Medical Encyclopedia Image www.nlm.nih.gov

Again, form follows function. The colon's main job is to reabsorb water and to absorb electrolytes, so it doesn't need villi to maximize absorption. Most nutrient absorption happens in the small intestine. Compared to the rifled barrel of the small intestine, the colon is a smooth-bore shotgun. It does have concertina-like folds called haustra, which act like baffles to slow down the fecal stream, to maximize water absorption.

If it's taken 6 hours for a Planter mouthful to make it this far, the military principle now kicks in – hurry up and wait – and it'll take another 18 hours to travel the last 6 feet (or 2 meters). The 6 or so quarts (or liters) of water we reabsorb are crucial for us to stay alive: if we lose this precious water through diarrhea, we die, as do thousands of 3rd World children each day because of contaminated drinking water.

Several bad things go wrong for Meaters and Junkers in their colons because of inadequate fiber and inadequate water. Instead of having large, soft fiber-packed stools in their colons, Meaters have small, dense, impacted, fiber-depleted, hard stools. Our muscular guts move our shit along by contracting in waves. This is called peristalsis, which means 'to wrap around.' Our gut walls contract in segments and this segmentation squeezes our poop to the next station, which in turn segments.

Constipation makes it harder for our guts to move our shit towards the exit.

Water is the true macro-nutrient… water and air. Without water we die, quickly. So our bodies will instruct our colons to extract every last drop it can, when it's running low. This sets up a vicious cycle. The more water we extract from our feces, the harder they become and the more difficult it becomes to move them, and the longer they stay in our colons. So we become more dehydrated and our bodies reabsorb more water, and so on.

The Appendix

There's a hollow, worm-like, six-inch long appendage hanging off the bottom of the ascending colon. It's called the appendix, and it's not an unnecessary relic – it's an integral part of our immune system and a source of healthy gut bacteria, from which we can recolonize our colons after a bout of antibiotics wipes them out.

When our colons become filled with hard and hard-to-budge feces, the opening to the appendix can become blocked with shit – especially as the pressure we exert when we're constipated is far higher than is healthy. Inflammation and infection can result, causing us to double over in pain, sometimes vomit, and then end up on a surgeon's table undergoing an appendectomy. This happens frequently to Meaters and Junkers; rarely to Planters.

Fruit is the natural antidote to constipation (and therefore to appendicitis). Besides being full of phytonutrients, fruits are full of water and fiber.

Our fecal stream now moves up the ascending colon, across the transverse, and down the descending colon. (Masseurs learn to rub up on the right-hand side of our abdomens, across, and then down on the left, so that they're not going against the flow.) Most of the pressure problems we experience show up in the last foot or so of our colons, 80% of them from the sigmoid on.

Diverticulosis ~ diverticulitis

When we're 'straining at stool,' we're pushing hard wide masses into a narrow rectal chamber, with an even narrower anus door at the far end. Something's gotta give... and sometimes the something is our intestinal wall. Little pockets get blown out at weak points, forming one diverticulum, several diverticula.

(**Polyps** are something else. They're bumps in the colon which develop out of epithelial cells and may be precursors to cancer. Berries are great at regressing what Meating causes.)

As we'd expect, these balloons can fill up with shit, become enflamed and infected. Diverticulosis has morphed into diverticulitis. If a diverticulum ruptures, it can spill shit out into our abdominal cavities, cause a condition of sepsis known as peritonitis and kill us.

Because of its location, diverticulitis is sometimes called 'left-sided appendicitis.' Diverticulitis and appendicitis happen in different parts of the colon, but they have the same Meater/Junker Eatiology.

Diverticula also set us up for colorectal cancer, which erases tens of thousands of Meaters and Junkers each year.

Meating and Junking → fiber and water deficiency → constipation → pressure "diseases" including diverticulitis → colorectal cancer.

Diverticular "disease" goes away on a Planter diet. The diverticula close up and wither away. Why would that surprise us? They're caused by Meating and Junking.

Hemorrhoids (Piles)

Not all things hemorrhoidal are bad: we have hemorrhoidal arteries and veins at the end of our poop chutes, around our anuses. When we apply pressure to hard turds in our rectums, we can cut off the blood flow in our hemorrhoidal veins. The back pressure causes them to bulge and become permanently varicose, or distended. We can get hemorrhoids internally or externally, or both, and sometimes the internal ones can 'prolapse' or fall out of our asses, requiring someone to stuff them back in again.

If we undergo any of the many procedures to remove piles, while continuing to Meat and Junk, we haven't done anything to remove the underlying cause… we haven't removed from our butts the things that wrecked 'em to begin with.

Hemorrhoids go away on a Planter diet.

Other pressure "diseases"

The Meater and Junker pressure "diseases" we've met so far are:

- Constipation
- hiatal hernia
- (appendicitis)
- diverticulosis and –itis; peritonitis
- ulcerative colitis
- hemorrhoids

The same high pressure mechanism causes varicose veins in our legs. Sometimes people exert so much pressure when they're straining to poop, they burst blood vessels… and aneurysms can be deadly. Colorectal cancer may follow from colitis.

Constipation can be lethal. Meaters and Junkers are full of it. Planters go with the flow…

Fiber and our gut flora

Planting activates our immune system in our intestines – alerting us to an encounter with the outside environment. And Planting beneficially interacts with our DNA to epigenetically up- and down-grade the expression of a multitude of genes. Planting does one other amazing thing: it creates and maintains the **organ** known as the **microbiome**. Synonyms are gut flora; beneficial bacteria; good bacteria, etc.

Our microbiome is what separates the amateur eaters from the pros. Here, for the umpteenth and last time in this book, is my role model, Dr. Michael Greger, on the subject of the microbiome:

715

"Health-promoting effects of our good bacteria include boosting our immune system, improving digestion and absorption, making vitamins, inhibiting the growth of potential pathogens, and keeping us from feeling bloated, but should bad bacteria take roost, they can produce carcinogens, putrefy protein in our gut, produce toxins, mess up our bowel function, and cause infections."

[See: http://nutritionfacts.org/video/microbiome-the-inside-story/]

Planting gives us a healthy microbiome organ that makes anti-cancer and anti-inflammatory substances like lignans, butyrate, acetate and propionate. A low level of butyrate in our colons, which is indicative of low fiber intake (i.e. a low level of Planting) and a depleted gut flora, is what starts the inflammatory cascade that leads to inflammatory bowel "diseases" such as ulcerative colitis and Crohn's "disease", and colorectal cancer. Planting, in effect, controls our enteric immune system, keeping it off and keeping us healthy when fiber is abundant; switching it on and attacking our guts when we're fiber-deficient. Meating and Junking are fiber-free disaster zones.

Fiber- and phytate-deficient Junking and Meating also provoke our microbiome to emit H_2S (because of the animal proteins) and to create TMAO (from the carnitine and choline), causing cancer and damaging our entire arterial tree.

Planting acknowledges that we – humans, that is – are outnumbered in our own bodies by bacteria, which live mainly in our colons. Not to feed them the fiber they thrive on is to be at war with ourselves. They're Planters; we're Planters. The only way to eat sanely and be well is to co-operate with the fellow components of our bodies.

Planting acknowledges that there's ~150 to 300 times more bacterial DNA in us than there is human DNA. Not to feed our bacteria the plants that benefit both 'us' and 'them' epigenetically is to be schizophrenic and sick. They are us; we are them; and we all thrive on the same whole plants.

I think that everyone would agree that taking antibiotics constantly would be terribly bad for our health, particularly for the health of our intestinal bacteria. But wait a moment… eating animals *is* like taking antibiotics all the time. Meating kills our beneficial bacteria in exactly the same way as taking antimicrobial drugs! The animals we eat *are* antibiotics.

The microbiome at the terminus of our digestive tracts is fed and nourished by Planting. It responds by feeding and nourishing us. To be a Meater or a

Junker is to live in a house divided and, as Jesus says: "If a house is divided against itself, that house cannot stand."

Jesus' code of ethics includes "Thou shalt not kill" and "Do unto others as you would have them do unto you," golden rules that ethical Planters abide by naturally on all levels.

The Buddha says that to be a Planter "is to step into the stream which leads to nirvana."

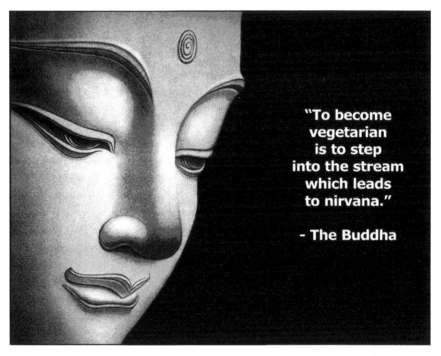

"To become vegetarian is to step into the stream which leads to nirvana."

- The Buddha

Prince Siddhartha. www.facebook.com/compassionateeaters/

In the Bhagavad Gita, Krishna says: "One who is not envious but who is a kind friend to all living entities… he is very dear to Me."

According to Isaiah, prophet to Muslims, Jews and Christians, Yahweh asks: "Of what use are all your sacrifices to Me? I have had enough of the roasted carcasses of Rams and of the fat of fattened Beasts. I take no pleasure in the blood of Calves, Lambs and Goats. When you spread out your hands, I close My eyes to you; despite however much you pray, I will not listen. Your hands are full of blood! Wash yourselves clean! Put away your misdeeds from before My eyes and stop doing evil."

Mahavira says: "Non–violence and kindness to living beings is kindness to oneself. For thereby one's own self is saved from various kinds of sins and resultant sufferings and is able to secure his own welfare."

And in the Quran we read: "There is not an animal on the earth, nor a flying creature on two wings, but they are people like unto you."

In our great religious teachings, the gut bone connects to the soul bone - animals aren't food; nor are they ours to think of as food.

~

Looking back

Okay, we've come to the end of Mr. Turd's wild ride through our colons. We need to go back now and study a few more of the trains Meating and Junking shunted into sidings or derailed along the tracks.

Fatty liver "disease"

As we saw earlier, alcohol, high-fructose, cholesterol and animal fats all contribute to fatty liver "disease". Healthy liver cells 'drop out' and gradually get replaced with fat cells. In time, scar tissue forms throughout the liver, and when the scar tissue contracts, the outer margins of the liver take on the scalloped appearance characteristic of cirrhosis. Now we have an irreversibly dysfunctional liver. Before that, Planting can reverse liver "disease". The liver is a marvel of regeneration, an absolute champion, when we feed it nothing but whole plant nutrients. Alcohol isn't a nutrient.

Kidney failure

'Meat + sweet' is what kills our kidneys. Industrial sugars, animal fats and animal proteins cause hyper-filtration and protein leakage. Planting keeps our kidneys healthy.

Gout and non-oxalate kidney stones are a product of eating industrial sugars and purines– Meating and Junking. Oxalate kidney stones form in the acid conditions Meating supplies – high-oxalate plants don't cause kidney stones.

Auto-immune conditions

For rheumatoid arthritis and other animal-borne auto-immune responses, let's go back a few steps to where the animals are first getting absorbed in our small intestine. The fatty acids have been released from the fats, and the amino acids have been semi-released from their proteins. Products of incomplete digestion, peptide chains are strings of amino acids that are still linked together. One such peptide in casein, the main protein in cow's milk, consisting of 17 amino acids, is identical to a peptide in the beta-cells of our pancreases, which are responsible for manufacturing insulin. In a friendly fire auto-immune attack, our immune system can wipe out the beta cells and cause irreparable type I diabetes.

Meating causes auto-immune responses. Therefore, animals cannot be food.

The Eatiology of most auto-immune "diseases" is similar: it's a reaction to the introduction of animal proteins which our bodies rightly consider to be inimical to our health. Lupus, MS and rheumatoid arthritis are Meater

719

conditions, symptoms not diseases, and they improve on a pure Planter diet.

Atherosclerosis & cardiovascular "disease"

Animal fats (and processed plant fats) provoke our livers to produce more cholesterol, to go along with the cholesterol we eat. Now, cholesterol, as we know by now, is a substance vital for good health, used in cell membranes and nerve cell sheaths, etc., but it's not a nutrient. We have zero need to eat cholesterol. Our bodies make it; always have, always will. In fact, cholesterol is another animal ingredient that provokes an immune response.

The beginning stage of atherosclerosis is when immune system cells called macrophages are galvanized into gobbling up cholesterol. The macrophages become full of cholesterol, they get sequestered in our arterial walls, becoming foam cells; the foam cells become fatty streaks; over time, our arteries become narrowed, enflamed and stiffened.

Anything we eat that causes an immune response in us has never been food. Both animal proteins and animal cholesterol disqualify animals on the ground that they cause our immune systems to try to destroy them

Animal proteins can do their damage relatively quickly, in weeks or months. Sadly, for us herbivores and the herbivores we eat, our auto-immune response to cholesterol (exacerbated by animal and junk fats) takes decades to manifest clinically. Sub-clinically, if we've been eating animals for years, we've all got heart and arterial "disease". Pure Planters are immune.

Atherosclerosis of the brain's arteries is what sets the stage for dementia, such as Alzheimer's, with animal-borne amyloidosis and metal deposits joining in the destruction.

Leaky gut

Saturated fats play another malefic role in the Meater Eatiology. They compromise the tight junctions of the enterocyte cell lining of our gut walls, allowing endotoxins – dead bacteria in animals – to penetrate where they don't belong and to enter our bloodstreams, causing endotoxemia – blood poisoning. With every bite we take, in microscopic amounts.

A crippling wave of 'stiffness' flows through our entire arterial tree after we eat a single high-fat meal, whether of animal or junk origin. BARTs (brachial artery reflex tests) show that it takes 6 or more hours for our arteries to return to baseline after a high-fat meal, by which time we're ready to repeat the procedure with more animals and junk.

Loosening our tight junctions, by allowing pathogens and large protein fragments free passage out of our guts, makes immune responses worse, and also makes Meaters more susceptible to allergic reactions such as hay fever and eczema (which they are). Meating causes a 'leaky gut,' a condition far more serious than its jokey-sounding name.

Over decades, atherosclerosis – an entirely Meater and Junker condition – causes insidious, unnoticed, under-diagnosed damage. Most people who die from heart attacks and strokes, do so suddenly, mysteriously, seemingly out of the blue. "But she looked so well…" "I can't believe it, he was so fit…" That's because even skinny, healthy-looking people can be fat on the inside, where it counts, in our heart and blood vessels. Like jogging guru Jim Fixx.

Cholesterol levels, as set by our foremost health authorities – read: Meaters – are criminally high. That's because healthy, low cholesterol levels are only possible with a pure Planter dietstyle. To be safe from heart attack and stroke, our total cholesterol levels need to be below 150 (3.9 in the UK) and LDL needs to be below 70-75 (1.9). That's it. Planters with cholesterol below those levels are "heart attack-proof," says Dr. Caldwell Esselstyn.

It doesn't matter whether we believe in cholesterol or not; cholesterol believes in us. It causes our immune systems to attack it when we eat or make it in excess. It's not food.

Saturated fats aren't the only culprit – fiber deficiency leads to a decrease in the number of good bacteria like *F. prausnitzii* in our colons, which leads in turn to a thinning of the protective mucous intestinal lining and damaged tight junctions, allowing pathogens to penetrate the gut wall, resulting in increased immune response and inflammation, and more inflammatory bowel "disease". Meating seems always to have redundant systems to cause harm.

Hypertension

Back to atherosclerosis… As Meating makes our arteries stiffer and narrower and less elastic, our blood pressure gradually rises. With narrower hose pipes, our hearts have to beat harder. Acute high blood pressure becomes permanent, chronic, even malignant hypertension, perhaps the best indicator we have for ill-health and imminent death; better even than high cholesterol levels. (High cholesterol shows that bad stuff could happen; hypertension shows it has already happened.)

Hypertension in turn sets us up for hemorrhagic stroke, while atherosclerosis is setting us up for ischemic stroke, two of our biggest killers… but these so-called diseases are all merely symptoms of the underlying Meating.

So, Meating causes inflammation, constriction of our arteries, elevated blood pressure… The narrowing of our arteries causes hypoperfusion in the tissues and organs our blood bathes: a reduction in blood flow, meaning a reduction in oxygen and nutrients.

Dementia

Our brains make up less than 2% of our body weight, but they receive about 20% of our blood flow. Hypoperfusion of our brains over time sets the stage for dementia. Atherosclerosis of the brain, caused by Meating, is what lays the table for Alzheimer's and other forms of dementia. At the same time that cholesterol is assaulting the blood-brain barrier and causing a 'leaky brain,' atherosclerosis is reducing brain blood supply, and increasing the possibility of infarctions and minor strokes. The other damage comes later, with misfolded animal proteins called amyloids, forming plaques and tangles, and metals like copper and iron complicating the mess that Meating started with coronary artery and carotid artery "disease".

Stiffened, diseased arteries – system-wide, not just in our hearts – can't dilate properly. Animals, deficient in nitrates, are unable to produce nitric oxide, the signaling molecule emitted by our endothelial cells to cause our vessels to dilate. Nitrates come from veggies, leafy greens in particular. Meaters are kept healthy to the extent we also include Planting.

Cancer

Meaters swallow excess hormones. Cow's milk in particular interferes with our own signaling systems. If we think of hormones as the chemical versions of our nervous system, carrying information and instructions from glands to muscles or other organs, would we eat a foreign species' nerves if they started ordering us around?

That's what we do when we drink animals' milk – we swallow their liquid nerves, and these alien hormones start ordering our bodies around. Milk is something we're only adapted to utilizing when we're infants: it's our growth-signaling stimulus. We have zero need of growth stimulus in adulthood. The hormones in milk – particularly the estrogens, some 15 of them – are what incite the "sexual cancers" in humans – cancers of breast, ovary, vagina, uterus and prostate.

Animal proteins are carcinogenic: when a load of animal proteins arrives in us, our livers – programmed to receive breast milk protein only in infancy – see protein bricks arrive and think, hell, it must be building time. So our livers start pumping out IGF-1, insulin-like growth factor, our human growth hormone.

Allied to the animal growth hormones we're Meating – plus the huge load of external chemical endocrine disruptors bio-magnified in animals – our own hormones + animal hormones + chemical hormone-like substances all promote cancer growth. Inappropriate stimulus of cell growth in us promotes cancer… And more rapid aging. The more hormones we eat (i.e., the more animals we eat), the more cancers we'll get. Cancer and rapid aging are symptoms of Meating.

Animal protein is carcinogenic. So too are the poultry and other oncogenic viruses that are in the animals. So too are the environmental chemicals that come packaged with the animals: the arsenic and lead and mercury and PCBS and phthalates and… and… and…

Cancer thrives on inflammation. Well, atherosclerosis does a good job of that, producing inflamed, ulcerated, pustular lesions in our arteries. Animal proteins cause inflammation. Animal fats promote inflammation through leaky guts. So does fiber deficiency. Animal blood iron (heme iron) causes inflammation. Arachidonic acid in animals causes inflammation. Neu5Gc causes so much inflammation it's known as the "inflammatory meat molecule." Meating initiates some tumors. The tumors that Meating causes use the inflammation Meating supplies to grow, and Meating promotes cancer, then makes tumors more invasive, causes angiogenesis in tumors (providing them with a blood supply), and finally promotes metastasis and spread to other parts of the body.

Obesity

Meating is also obesogenic: it makes us fat. So too is Junking. Planters are the only sector of society that's not overweight. Meating and Junking are both nutrient-poor and energy-dense. It's vice versa for Planting. Already too rich in calories, Meating also provides chemical and biological obesogens that make us fatter – endocrine-disrupting pollutants and obesogenic viruses, found most often in chickens. Meating even provides us with infectobesity – obesity as an animal virus-borne "disease". (I find this concept astonishing.)

Obese people's fat cells create estrogens of their own, thereby completing the circle of why obesity and cancer are so strongly linked. The spillover effect causes obese people to constantly have high levels of circulating blood fats, even when not eating much food, completing the circle of why obesity and insulin resistance go together; their partnership sometimes called diabesity. These are Meater and Junker conditions, not Planter.

Lung health

When we eat lots of animal proteins, our stomachs secrete obscene amounts of acid. Acid reflux can cause problems to the esophagus, as we saw earlier. In our mouths, the acid can eat away the enamel on our teeth and can cause a persistent cough and damage to our throats - giving us a hoarse, Lauren Bacall-like voice - and chronic exposure of our lungs to acid can lead to asthma and even emphysema.

The high sulfur content of animal proteins is what gives Meaters their characteristic bad breath, redolent of rotten eggs, and also their repellent, meaty body odor. Occidental Meaters smell rank to the Orientals who're still eating their traditional low-animal diets (and to Planters eating their traditional no-animal diets). Uber-meaters on ketogenic diets also exhale ketones, giving them 'rotten apple breath' to go along with the stench of putrescent eggs.

Aging

Methionine and leucine, two amino acids found predominantly in animals, a surfeit of calories (found in both Meating and Junking) and a generally acidified, oxidized and inflammatory state are the main reasons we age prematurely. (There's a very lengthy description of aging in Part 1B (Mechanisms).)

All of these Eatiological mechanisms are in play at the same time, affecting every single part of our bodies, sapping our immune systems and making us more susceptible to illness.

The Meater abyss

The Meater pit is bottomless. Just when we think we've scraped the bottom with animals-as-food, new research comes in to add another layer of evidence of their anti-food nature. Every month I read papers showing things like... Animal proteins overload our kidneys and cause them to decline in function. Animal fats cause fatty liver "disease" and set us up for hepatitis and liver failure or cancer. Animal arachidonic acid causes inflammation in our brains. Animal casomorphins, made from the beta-casein in cows' milk, kill infants via crib death (sudden infant death syndrome or SIDS). The hormones in milk cause acne, another biomarker for heart "disease" and early death. The HAs and PAHs that form when we incinerate animals cause cancer. And on, and on, with never any peer-reviewed science to show a benefit of Meating. Plenty out there in the blogosphere and from non-researchers with books to sell to the credulous; none done by reputable scientists untainted by industry money. None. Ever. How can I be so sure? Because it's not possible - animals aren't food.

Death

With Meaters and Junkers, it's a race… It's only a matter of chance which symptom of Meating and Junking gets to the finishing line first: will we die of a heart attack, or will the piece of atheroma that breaks off lodge in our brains and kill us with a stroke? Or will the hypoxia brought about by atherosclerosis cause a tumor, which meatastasizes into our bone marrow and does us in, before our liver shrivels and quits? It doesn't matter what the coroner writes in the book – Sudden Cardiac Death, stroke, malignant neoplasm, hepatitis – the real ur-causes of death are Meating and Junking.

Animals themselves, via their three main inbuilt mechanisms of atherosclerosis, oncogenesis and auto-immunity, degrade our systems, slowly sickening and killing us.

Animals introduce most of the chemical pollutants, which we then need to detoxify and expel; sometimes they sicken and kill us.

Animals introduce most of the pathogens, which we then need to combat and kill; sometimes they win, and they sicken and kill us.

Animals are almost entirely deficient in beneficial nutrients, while being saturated with lethal ingredients and overly-endowed with energy and sulfurous proteins.

It's a sad fact that our constitutions are too resilient for our own good. If the animals we eat were to incite more violent and acute symptoms in us instead of the insidious chronic, almost invisible symptoms that they do, we'd all be better off. Non-human animals would be too. Our bodies' resistance to the daily onslaught of Meating is nothing short of miraculous.

725

"What a piece of work is a [hu]man!
How noble in reason, how infinite in faculty!
In form and moving how express and admirable!
In action how like an angel, in apprehension how like a god!
The beauty of the world. The paragon of animals.
And yet, to me, what is this quintessence of dust?
Man delights not me. No, nor woman neither, …"

Not when we betray our angelic natures by ignorantly stuffing ourselves full of the bodies of dead animals. We are not paragons then; we are not then like a god. When we eat animals, we become fallen angels. Then we're beneath bestial, for every beast knows what is and what isn't food.

Except humans.

As smart as we are, we're exceptionally stupid when it comes to eating, a most basic of animal functions.

We Americans in particular *are* exceptional. Not because outdated or silly ideas like Manifest Destiny or "the end of history" made us so; because of our Meater and Junker mal-nutrition. We're exceptionally ignorant about food and, as a result, we're exceptionally fat and diseased. We spend more on healthcare than the next gazillion countries put together [numbers can be numb-ers – they numb us] and still we have worse health than 30-odd countries, coming in roughly the same as Cuba, a country we've embargoed for a half-century, peevishly driving their economy into the rubble because they chose to be free of us. And yet, despite their economic disadvantages, they have good health… partly because they eat so many plants and so few animals, and partly because there's a shortage of pharmaceutical drugs. Both are unforeseen benefits of our suffocating their industrialization.

Meating is what harms us; Planting is what makes us whole.

We can only become "noble in reason" again, and "infinite in faculty" when we re-learn how to eat. The scientific evidence is in: animals aren't food.

I hope this brief synopsis of a Meater meal serves to show how dangerous Meating and Junking are. Obviously, I've just pointed out the molehill – there's far more going on underground than I've had the skills or the space to describe. But you get the drift...

Meating kills, dear hearts. Animals aren't food. Should I say it again? Ah, what the heck… Animals aren't food.

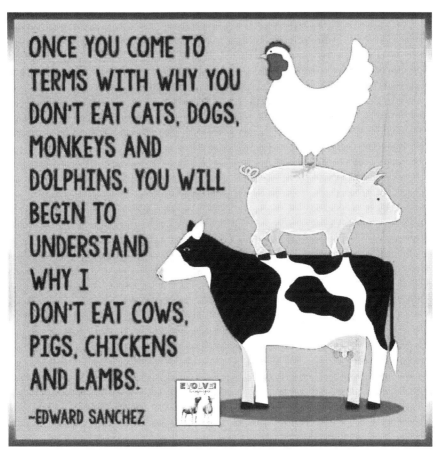

Edward Sanchez quote. Image, with thanks: Evolve! Campaigns

On Silver Bullets & Coffin Nails

Here's a list of ten silver bullets that shoot down the ghoul of Meating; or ten coffin nails that seal the lid of the gruesome, abusive, pointless practice. These are ten truths that, each on their own, should be enough to show that animals aren't food. When taken in their totality they make it certain that they're not. Certain, that is, to eaters who're willing to follow the Eatiology and nothing but the Eatiology to its logical conclusion.

#1 is **animal protein**. Animal protein causes a whole slew of auto-immune responses in those who eat it, such as type I diabetes, rheumatoid arthritis and multiple sclerosis. *They're* animals; *we're* animals; our bodies can't tell the difference. Foods don't cause auto-immune responses.

#2 is **animal protein**. Eating animal proteins after infancy, when we should have been weaned off animals, signals our bodies to release IGF-1, thus initiating cancer and speeding up aging.

#3 is **heme iron**. Our bodies lack a regulatory mechanism for inflammatory heme iron. Animal blood is thus "evolutionarily novel" to us, still unprocessable after millions of years.

#4 is **cholesterol**. Atherosclerosis is a condition found naturally only in herbivores. We get atherosclerosis when we eat animals. Therefore, we are herbivores. Atherosclerosis is our bodies' immune response to cholesterol, potentiated by animal and junk fats. Anything that causes an immune response isn't food.

#5 is **Neu5Gc**, another animal component that causes an immune response in us, leads to a cascade of inflammation, and conditions that thrive in inflammatory conditions, such as cancer. Arachidonic acid and alpha-gal, also found only in animals, are other similar examples of Meater silver bullets, but I throw them in here for free.

#6 is our **small intestines' immune function**. Even though Meating provides more than 90% of the toxic load of hundreds of CONSTITUENTS, PATHOGENS and CONTAMINANTS, the small gut's immune system is activated especially by cruciferous plants, proving that plants formed the overwhelming majority of the diets of proto-humans, and, probably, that our remote ancestors ate nothing but plants.

#7 is our **colonic gut flora**. Though made up of trillions of separate micro-organisms, our gut flora is tantamount to a separate human organ. Meaters have high-sulfur gut flora that produce H_2S and TMAO, with a resulting torrent of "disease", while Planters' gut bacteria produce health-promoting butyrate, acetate and propionate. Eating high-fiber whole plants keeps our immune systems well-calibrated, and us free from inflammatory "diseases".

#8 is **zeaxanthin+lutein**. These plant pigments are our eye pigments. When we eat leafy green vegetables, these two phytonutrients make a beeline for the retinas and lenses of our eyes, and take up residence there. They become us; we are them. (Miraculous chlorophyll, a blood tonic and carcinogen interceptor, is another Planter silver bullet freebie.)

#9 is **dietary intervention studies**, the gold standard of practical nutrition science. Instead of looking at a single variable such as cholesterol, as reductionists are wont to do, when we change people's entire diet to Pure Planting, conditions such as type II diabetes, heart "disease", prostate cancer, auto-immune conditions... aging!... slow down, stop, and sometimes even reverse. Lifestyle practitioners such as Nathan Pritikin, Roy Swank, Walter Kempner, Dean Ornish, Caldwell Esselstyn Jr., Neal Barnard, Brenda Davis and John McDougall have proved this over and over again, for fifty years and more.

#10 is the **Adventist Studies**. These are like dietary intervention studies at the population level, and they show that the longest-lived people ever studied are the vegans among the 7th Day Adventist community in and around Loma Linda, CA. Outliving the general populace by 10 to 14 years, exercising, non-smoking, non-drinking, non-Junking Loma Linda vegans are the longest-lived people ever recorded. They never eat animals.

With the gradual addition of animals to their diet, Adventists, just like the rest of us, become, by quantum leaps, fatter, more diabetic, more osteoporotic and hypertensive, more heart-diseased and shorter-lived. The Proof is in the Planter Pudding.

Taken as a group of ten inescapable facts about Meating, these final ten truths are the nails in the Meater coffin:

Animals aren't food.

~

The Pointlessness of Meating

If I've done my job, we now agree that animals and other junk aren't food.

If animals aren't food, isn't much of what we do pointless?

We smash down rain forests – the lungs of our planet – so we can eat cheap non-foods.

We strip-mine our oceans so we can eat the non-foods we quarry there.

In order to feed the animals we eat, we pour gigatons of chemicals on our land, which end up killing our waterways and oceans.

We give massive subsidies to non-food farmers to grow "food" that kills us, and a mere pittance to food farmers who heal us.

Why Does a Salad Cost More Than a Big Mac?

Federal Subsidies for Food Production, 1995-2005*   **Federal Nutrition Recommendations**

Vegetables, Fruits: 0.37%

Nuts and Legumes: 1.91%

Sugar, Oil, Starch, Alcohol: 10.69%

Grains: 13.23%

Meat, Dairy: 73.80%

Sugar, Oil, Salt (use sparingly)

Protein: includes meat, dairy, nuts, and legumes (6 servings)

Vegetables, Fruits (9 servings)

Grains (11 servings)

Why does a salad cost more than a Big Mac? Source: PCRM

With the US government, money speaks louder than words: 85% of subsidies go to Meating and Junking, 15% to food.

We give 85% of agricultural subsidies to the non-food sector that causes 90% of our health care costs, which are bankrupting us, as families and as a nation. Our Meater government gives our money to their Meater cronies

730

who're killing us, and when we inevitably become sick it gives our money to their pals in the insurance and medical industries that refuse to heal us with plants.

We feed most of the healing plants we grow to non-human animals that sicken us. Especially corn, even though cattle can't digest it.

We feed tons of antimicrobial drugs to animals so that they can grow faster; so our children may die quicker when the drugs become impotent.

We spend billions on drugs to counter our own impotence, instead of stopping eating animals, which is what makes us impotent.

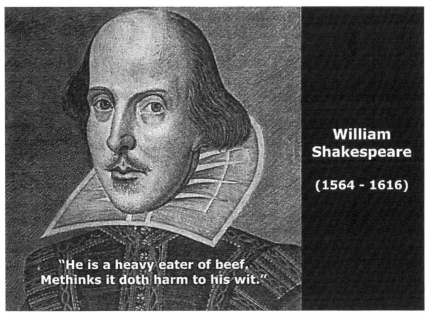

William
Shakespeare

(1564 - 1616)

"He is a heavy eater of beef.
Methinks it doth harm to his wit."

Billy Waggledagger, as my mother Fay used to call him....
www.facebook.com/compassionateeaters/

We rent out vast tracts of public land to non-food farmers at pennies on the dollar.

We have a government department that kills all the wildlife that competes with non-food farmers on their cheap public land. Orwell would have approved of its doublespeak name – The Department of Wildlife Services.

We have states in which it's illegal to "disparage" "foods" even though they're not plants and, therefore, not foods.

Our federal government has passed an Animal Enterprise Terrorism Act to protect animal wrongs activists, or animal abusers perpetrating "generally accepted practices," from the sane indignation of animal rights activists.

We have states which will jail us for taking photos of the wretched places where they disassemble animals to produce non-foods.

We have a Department of Agriculture that subsidizes, publicizes and promotes non-foods, even though 'truth in advertising' laws don't allow them to call these products 'healthy' or 'nutritious' or even 'safe.'

We have 5-yearly Nutrition Guidelines Committees, staffed by industry-owned Junkers and Meaters, that kill us by recommending we eat non-foods; those at the pinnacle of their "Food" Pyramids or on MyPlates. (To show a glass of milk next to MyPlate is asinine.)

We have a CDC that purports to control and prevent diseases, while remaining ignorant of Planting's ability to control and prevent "disease", and ignorant of the prime and choice roles Meating plays in the Eatiology of infections.

We have an NIH that tells us such bizarre rubbish as "Most adults do not get enough dairy products." Unbelievably crass, this nightmarish nutrition advice comes from the NIH's National Institute on Aging.

We have a Food and Drug Administration that's all about drugs (to combat the effects of Meating) and nothing about foods (which naturally avoid the effects of Meating).

As Wendell Berry says: "People are fed by the food industry, which pays no attention to health, and are treated by the health industry, which pays no attention to food."

We have a government that's besieged by armies of lobbyists of special interest groups, whose interests aren't special to the overwhelming majority of Americans, who just aren't special enough. The siege analogy is wrong, for the armies are ensconced within the citadel. We're on the outside.

We have a supreme court that's enshrined the rights of corporations, without defining any of their responsibilities beyond profit-making. While corporations remain "legal persons" and aren't constrained in the amounts of money they can contribute to election campaigns, we're all in trouble. The money will continue to flow into the pockets of elected officials who care nothing for public opinion or the truth about food.

We spend far many more billions of dollars on advertising and phony scientific studies for non-foods than it costs to produce them. Just as the tobacco companies used to do. In fact, they're the same people: the companies themselves and their gun-for-hire scientific and PR assassins. "Doubt is their product."

The parent company of Registered Dieticians – The Academy of Dietetics and Nutrition (AND) – is a morally bankrupt, quasi-owned subsidiary of Big Animal, Big Chemical and Big Junk, forced by their sell-out to their corporate sponsors such as Monsanto, Pepsi, Coke, Lay's and MacDonald's to tell us such preposterous whoppers as "There are no good or bad foods."

We eat more animals than any human population that's ever existed. And more junk.

Because we're suffering from Meater and Junker mal-nutrition, other dominoes fall…

We're the fattest, sickest people who've ever lived.

70% of us are taking at least one medication and 10%, five or more.

With 2.5 million Americans in jail, we have the largest prison population that's ever existed; many incarcerated for victimless crimes… drug crimes which I (as an ex-addict) think stem from our greatest addiction of all: eating animals.

We're a violent people, made so by our Meating.

We have as many guns in the US as we have people, which doesn't bother me as much as the fact that we're Meaters and nothing loath to use our guns on other animals and other people. Planters don't kill animals, either non-human or human.

We have the largest land, sea, air and special forces the world has ever seen. We have five thousand military bases in the continental USA and another thousand overseas in more than 150 countries. Not including its sand castle atolls in the South China Sea, China has one overseas base. Russia has three.

We kidnap our perceived enemies [rendition], smuggle them into prisons [black sites] and then torture them [extraordinary interrogation techniques], even though we know that the intel gained from torture is useless. Guantanamo remains open for business.

We have thousands of drones that patrol the skies ceaselessly, piloted by Meaters half a world away, murdering some perceived enemies, while murdering many more unlucky bystanders, who we shrug off as "collateral damage." We have a president who personally selects targets for drone strikes, including US citizens, as if he's playing video games, and to hell with the 9 unlucky passersby who don't vote.

We kill 100 billion land animals and maybe a trillion sea creatures each year… collateral damage to our societal ignorance about what is and what isn't food.

We have ten or eleven aircraft carrier groups that patrol the oceans continuously; each with enough firepower to destroy entire nations. We do this to maintain a constant flow of energy, which is the lifeblood of Empire, and then we squander the energy on inefficient cars and an inefficient, insane way of eating.

We put more energy into rearing non-foods than we get back from eating them. We transport some of the things we eat thousands of miles before eating them.

We may generate up to half of greenhouse gases in putting dead animals on our plates. For our eating pleasure, almost 100 million cattle share America with 320 million humans, and each of those animals contributes (fill in a numb-er (say) thirty) times more environmental waste than a human animal.

We use [fill in a numb-er, say 2 or 10 or 20] times as much water to grow one non-food meal than a food meal with the same energy content.

And our drinkable water is ~~running out~~ being pumped out; the high mountain snowpacks are dwindling; the glaciers are melting; the prehistoric aquifers are being siphoned dry, and the water tables are plummeting. We're flinging the water out carelessly on the land to grow crops to feed to animals, and then it disappears into the salt seas, lost for human use.

We use (say) 10 times as much fuel; 10 times as much land; 10 times as many inputs such as poisonous energy-dense fertilizers and pesticides for growing genetically modified crops to feed the animals we eat, compared to Planting.

In effect, it takes the food of 10 to 20 Planters to feed 1 Meater. In effect, a population of 320 million Meater Americans is eating the food of between 3.2 and 6.4 billion Planter humans. Or only 1.6 billion. What does it matter?

We're still eating way more than our fair share. (Perhaps that's the freedom we're hated for, little Georgie Jr?)

We're eating our planet to death, so that we can eat ourselves to death with non-foods.

We 1st Worlders are malnourished with too much, while the remaining 80% of humanity survive on our leftovers, and at least a billion people are malnourished because they have too little. When we eat ourselves to death on animals, we're also eating to death those to whom we've denied grains by feeding them to animals who can't digest them.

In the words of my beloved Thay… Thich Nhat Hanh:

> "Every day forty thousand children die in the world for lack of food. We who overeat in the West, who are feeding grains to animals to make meat, are eating the flesh of these children."

All pointless… Because animals aren't food, dear gorgeous people.

It's not too late to wake up.

To be a Planter is to be awake and on the side of the angels.

~

Meating and Earth's Climate

Near the end of the 20th Century, well-known Cornell ecologist David Pimentel told us: "If all the grain currently fed to livestock in the United States were consumed directly by people, the number of people who could be fed would be nearly 800 million." It's probably a billion people by now.

Cornell Chronicle Aug. 7, 1997.
http://www.news.cornell.edu/stories/1997/08/us-could-feed-800-million-people-grain-livestock-eat

Meanwhile, Meater climate change activist Bill McKibben (founder of 350.org) wants us to lower atmospheric carbon dioxide to 350 parts per million, while he continues to scarf down liverwurst sandwiches, as he does in *The End of Nature* (the book that first alerted us to climate change).

Al Gore, another well-known climate change activist, found Meating too inconvenient a truth to mention in his documentary, *An Inconvenient Truth*.

As film director James Cameron says, it's not possible to be an effective environmentalist *and* a Meater, Bill and Al. It's one or the other. And if you're a Planter now, Al, you need to bite the bullet and include Planting in your message – it's far more effective than keeping our car tires pumped up or installing special light bulbs or driving hybrid cars.

Actually, our inability to reach anything near peak performance while we carry on Meating is true of all occupations. It goes for conservationists and ecologists and ethologists and anthropologists and game park rangers and oceanographers and marine biologists (as confirmed by the wonderful Sylvia Earle - "There's still time, but not a lot, to turn things around"), and it goes for veterinarians and nutritionists and dieticians and chefs and physicians and public health officials and farmers and scientists and hospital administrators and caterers and athletes and bodybuilders and doulas and spiritual guides of all denominations… and… and… and… especially economists (still seeking infinite growth on our finite planet).

We only become truly human when we stop eating an inhuman diet of animals and junk. It's the difference between being easily, unconsciously humane and trying to make conscious humane choices; the difference between unconscious mastery and conscious incompetence.

To try to be healthy while continuing to Junk and Meat is to pee into a hurricane – there's bound to be lots of blowback.

Hospitals selling McDonald's "food," schools using milk or egg board indoctrination materials, alphabet-soup governmental organizations such as the CDC, the USDA, the NIH, the EPA and FDA, sundry organizations devoted to individual maladies like heart "disease," diabetes and cancer … all of these groups are complicit in keeping Meating unobjectionable. All of them should get their acts together, for the sake of our individual and societal health.

When it comes to planetary health, Meating is just as culpable. Here's some info about greenhouse gases from the Center for Climate and Energy Solutions, which shows that, while eliminating industrial coolants and refrigerants etc. is necessary, the best way to stop and reverse climate change is by eradicating animal agriculture.

Greenhouse Gas	Chemical Formula	Anthropogenic Sources	Atmospheric Lifetime[1] (years)	GWP[2] (100 Year Time Horizon)
Carbon Dioxide	CO_2	Fossil-fuel combustion, Land-use conversion, Cement Production	~100[1]	1
Methane	CH_4	Fossil fuels, Rice paddies, Waste dumps	12[1]	25
Nitrous Oxide	N_2O	Fertilizer, Industrial processes, Combustion	114[1]	298
Tropospheric Ozone	O_3	Fossil fuel combustion, Industrial emissions, Chemical solvents	hours-days	N.A.
CFC-12	CCL_2F_2	Liquid coolants, Foams	100	10,900
HCFC-22	CCl_2F_2	Refrigerants	12	1,810
Sulfur Hexaflouride	SF_6	Dielectric fluid	3,200	22,800

Main greenhouse gases.
Source: http://www.c2es.org/facts-figures/main-ghgs

We see that the GWPs (global warming potentials) of the Meater greenhouse gases – methane and nitrous oxide (CH_4 and N_2O) – are 25 and 298 respectively. That is, they are 25 and 298 times more damaging than CO_2, the benchmark gas. [Or 78 or 12 or whatever… a *lot*…]

Removing the nitrous oxide is equivalent to removing more than three hundred times as much CO_2, because it persists 1.14 times as long.

Removing methane has a double benefit. While it's 'only' 25 times more potent than CO_2, its 'atmospheric lifetime' is a mere 12 years, in comparison to CO_2's 100. So, over the course of a century, removing one molecule of methane is equivalent to removing $25 \times 100 \div 12 = 208$ molecules of CO_2.

Plus, when we look at the next table we see that methane is the gas that has built up the most in the troposphere since the industrial revolution began:

	Pre-1750 Tropospheric Concentration[3] (parts per billion)	Current Tropospheric Concentration[4] (parts per billion)
Carbon Dioxide	280,000[5]	388,500[6]
Methane	700[7]	1,870 / 1,748[8]
Nitrous Oxide	270[9]	323 / 322[8]
Tropospheric Ozone	25	34
CFC-12	0	.534 / .532[6]
HCFC-22	0	.218 / .194[10]
Sulfur Hexaflouride	0	.00712 / .00673[3, 10]

Changes in tropospheric concentrations of greenhouse gases.
Source: http://www.c2es.org/facts-figures/main-ghgs

While CO_2 levels have gone up 38.75% since 1750, N_2O levels have gone up 19.63%. But methane levels have catapulted up by 167.14%... Atmospheric methane is 2 and 2/3 times as bad now as it was back then, plus methane is 25 times as harmful as carbon dioxide.

Methane is the main climate changer; not CO_2, and not the CFCs, the HCFCs or the sulfur hexafluoride, which have all gone up infinitely, because they didn't exist in 1750, but which we produce in much smaller quantities.

Thank heavens for that. What good news.

Why? Because:

1. Methane is the most harmful greenhouse gas;
2. Confined animals are the biggest source of methane, and the one most easily stopped;

738

3. Animals aren't food, so (2) is unnecessary (even suicidal);
4. Methane survives in the atmosphere for only 12 years; so
5. If we stop creating MEAThane, we can limit climate change in just over a decade, and perhaps even stop it.

The best way to prevent climate change – now, before the frozen northern tundra releases its giga-load of methane – is to stop eating animals.

There's no other strategy that comes close to the effectiveness of this one (which also happens to be the healthiest choice for us): we'll preserve the Earth as we know it, when we stop killing other animals and ourselves.

Not to mention the metaphysical liberation and the spiritual joy that become possible when we stop the screams of the tens of billions of land animals we kill each year, which I imagine resounding through space instead of the Music of the Spheres or Johann Strauss's 'Beautiful Blue Danube,' which played during the unforgettable scene in *2001: A Space* Odyssey in which Discovery One glides out past Jupiter.

This is why angels don't like to come here any more – they have sensitive hearing and they can't bear the cacophony of animal bellowing emanating from Earth. Have you seen any angels lately? I haven't. (Do angels have delicate, hollow bones like birds? Why are their wings and arms separate structures?)

Just as Planters aren't serial killers, neither are we the main cereal consumers – Meaters top those lists. The Cornell Chronicle article about David Pimentel, quoted earlier, says: "From one ecologist's perspective, the American system of farming grain-fed livestock consumes resources far out of proportion to the yield, accelerates soil erosion, affects world food supply and will be changing in the future."

The very near future.

Either we change the climate now, by stopping Meating, or Meating will continue to change our climate and stop us. The planet will be just fine; we may not be so lucky.

Our recognition that animals aren't food is crucial to our species' future wellbeing. The World Health Organization acknowledged this on 26 October 2015, when they confirmed that processed animals are Group 1 carcinogens – on a par with arsenic, asbestos, alcohol and cigarette smoke – and that less-processed animals cause a lower level of carcinogenicity.

"Overall, the Working Group classified consumption of processed meat as "carcinogenic to humans" (Group 1) on the basis of sufficient evidence for colorectal cancer... The Working Group classified consumption of red meat as "probably carcinogenic to humans" (Group 2A)."

See: Véronique Bouvard, Dana Loomis, Kathryn Z Guyton, Yann Grosse, Fatiha El Ghissassi, Lamia Benbrahim-Tallaa, Neela Guha, Heidi Mattock, Kurt Straif, on behalf of the International Agency for Research on Cancer Monograph Working Group. Carcinogenicity of consumption of red and processed meat. *Lancet Oncol* 2015 Published Online October 26, 2015 http://dx.doi.org/10.1016/ S1470-2045(15)00444-1

(Look, we've known this for decades – while vested interests have fought us tooth and nail, just as they did with asbestos and smoking, using the same mercenary White Coats to confuse matters – but it's great that our most authoritative public health organizations are now stating the facts. The WHO publishing in *The Lancet*... it doesn't get much better than that.)

This gives us a wonderful opportunity to continue to eat fewer animals (the way the industrialized world has been doing for the last decade) and to stop the acceleration of Meating that's happening among the nouveau riche, promoted by external Western corporations who also pushed smoking and banned pesticides there when sales fell off back at home.

For our own personal health and for the health of our planetary home, there is no more important realization:

Animals aren't food.

~

The Good News

It's not all doom and gloom. There is good news. Great news, in fact.

Planting fixes just about everything that ails us.

It restores us to health.

It's the best weight management program around, without an Oprah, yoyo effect. It's permanent.

It removes our most fundamental addiction, making it easier for other addictions to melt away.

It restores our sanity. It makes us less violent, more serene.

It restores us to our true selves, removing the cognitive dissonance which blinds us when we say we love animals, while we eat them. We can only truly love animals when we're Planters.

When our circle of compassion lassos all species, and encircles even Meater humans, then we become more embracing, less chauvinist, less bellicose.

If we need to love ourselves before we can love others, we love ourselves best by being Planters.

Planting restores Nature, and allows us to relax into the food web, instead of clawing our way to the top of an imaginary, self-imposed food chain.

It makes wild animals numinous again; if they're not food, then they're holy. Precious; not trophies, not game, not meat.

Planting solves the problems of peak oil and how to feed a growing world population. It's an antidote to consumerism.

It helps stop climate change, whether we believe in it or not.

It stops deforestation and soil erosion and desertification.

It stops the acidification and eutrophication of our seas and lakes and streams.

It preserves the ancient water in our aquifers.

It preserves the ancient sunlight, our dwindling hydrocarbon reserves.

It preserves the quality of our air.

It would stop the current great extinction event, the only one in billions of years perpetrated by one species upon millions of others.

It stops the extinction of the antibiotics which have been such a boon to us, and whose loss may condemn millions to death in a bleak future.

It stops the development and spread of zoönotic plagues, from hyper-confined non-humans to hyper-confined humans.

When we stop our pointless eating of animals, we heal our most basic wounds: our estrangement from the other sentient beings with whom we share this beautiful blue world, and our estrangement from our best selves.

Meating was our opportunistic past…

Junking is our ignorant present…

Planting is our beautiful future.

I hope to see you there.

~

Acknowledgments

I wouldn't have been able to write this book were it not for the work of the extraordinary Dr. Michael Greger, who's done more than any other person to bring the intricacies of nutrition science to a lay audience. His website – www.nutritionfacts.org – is a resource without peer. I urge you to seek it out, if you don't already know it. I'll go so far as to call it a service to humanity. It's totally free, a 501c3 nonprofit charity supported by donations, and I encourage anyone who benefits from its brilliance to contribute.

I also recommend Dr. Greger's groundbreaking new book: *How Not to Die: Discover the Foods Scientifically Proven to Prevent and Reverse Disease.* Definitive.

Every year Dr. Greger "reads through every issue of every English-language nutrition journal in the world so [we] don't have to." His annual, hour-long presentation previewing his work of the year to come is an eagerly awaited event, and the back editions can be found on nutritionfacts.org or YouTube. Besides being densely informative, they're entertaining (and wickedly funny!)

(His jest that "if there's one thing we know about hot dog eaters, it's that they're picky about what goes in their food" always cracks me up.)

On Mondays, Wednesdays and Fridays of each week, Dr. Greger posts a short new video on an aspect of nutrition and health that he and his team have gleaned from their reading. All back numbers are archived and efficiently searchable by keyword, of which there are more than a thousand.

On Tuesdays and Thursdays, Dr. Greger posts an article. He lists all the sources he cites in his videos and articles, and clicking the hyperlinks takes us straight to the relevant papers, in such prestigious journals as the *New England Journal of Medicine, The Lancet,* the *American Journal of Clinical Nutrition* and hundreds of others, some quite obscure, so we can read and verify the primary materials for ourselves, if we so wish.

I did so wish, and it was Dr. Greger who inspired my nutrition education and the writing of this book. If I've quoted Dr. Greger or nutritionfacts.org a hundred times in this book, I wouldn't be surprised. I can't claim to have read all the papers he's referenced, but I do have a burgeoning collection of "landmark" masterpieces such as Dr. Dean Ornish et al's 1990 *Lancet* paper which first proved that a pure plant diet can reverse heart "disease". I date

the beginning of modern lifestyle medicine from the day – 21 July 1990 –
on which Dr. Ornish and his co-workers posed the question: "Can lifestyle
changes reverse coronary heart disease?"

The answer was a resounding "yawp" of a yes. At that time, modern
medicine had degenerated into mere symptom management, via chemistry,
radiation and surgery (where it still languishes, for the most part). Then
Ornish showed us that healing *is* possible, not by suppressing symptoms,
but by removing root causes. And the way we heal is through Right
Nutrition… through Planting. And Planting removes multiple, multiple
maladies, as I've shown, as much through the life-affirming benefits of
Planting as through ending the habitual, repetitive injuries of Meating and
Junking.

I have any number of Planter heroes. Those with whom I've studied, and
through whom I've gained some modest accreditation in nutrition science
and dietstyle counseling, include Prof. T. Colin Campbell of Cornell,
eCornell and the T. Colin Campbell Foundation; Dr. Neal Barnard of
PCRM, Food for Life and The George Washington University; The
Plantrician Project; Dr. John McDougall of *The Starch Solution*, Dr.
McDougall's Health and Medical Center and the McDougall Research &
Education Foundation; Mary-Ann and Mark Shearer of The Natural Way,
and Will Tuttle, PhD, author of *The World Peace Diet – Eating for Spiritual
Health and Social Harmony* [required reading for all eaters everywhere,
everywhen], and leading light of Prayer Circle for Animals and the World
Peace and Yoga Jubilee … astonishingly wonderful humans, all.

I owe you all a debt of gratitude for the decades of work you've put into
making our world a healthier, happier, holier place. Kudos to you all, and to
all my fellow Planters, those of us who're already here and those of us
who're yet to be.

~

"What's next?" and "Staying in touch"

One of the worst disease vectors infecting our planet today is a group of individuals who, for reasons best known to themselves, are spreading deadly low-carb and paleo diets. I've made it my life's mission to out these propagandists, confusionists and denialists for the scientific frauds they are.

Because animals aren't food, as I've just demonstrated via hundreds of animal components, harmful mechanisms, pathogens, contaminants and deficiencies, the Low-Carb Bullshit Artists are forced to use any means, usually foul, to whitewash Meating. I hope you'll join me in my next book, **The Low-Carb Bullshit Artists Are Lying Us to Death**, which details the many ways these un-empathic, even psychopathic, surreal killers go about their slimy business. [See pp. 791 - 822, About my next book.]

Why Animals Aren't Food consumed five years of my life. I looked everywhere for a compilation of the science showing the harmfulness of eating animals, but there wasn't one, so I realized I'd have to write it myself.

Now, when I'm not busy revising this book and writing the next, I'm going to ramp up my first love, which is public speaking. I really enjoy thinking and talking about nutrition. Interacting with people about how to eat is what really blows my hair back - what there is of it - and it's rewarding to coax an audience into appreciating the glories of Planting and the miseries of Meating.

I also enjoy coaching a select few motivated over-achievers, helping them to gain even more edginess, the Planter way.

Nutrition science is only now entering its Planter Renaissance after the Meater Middle Ages, and there's a ferment of Planter nutrition science constantly brewing, so if you enjoyed <u>Why Animals Aren't Food</u> please go to *WAAF*'s Facebook page at https://www.facebook.com/whyanimalsarentfood/, and if you Like the page, you'll receive the updates I plan to make in the future.

The address for the *WAAF* website is <u>www.whyanimalsarentfood.com</u>.

I manage two other Facebook pages besides *WAAF*'s. One is a community page called <u>Compassionate Eaters</u> and it contains images of and sayings by inspirational vegan and near-vegan role models down the ages, to help keep vegans inspired and proud of our awesome lineage, stretching back to

Pythagoras and beyond. You can find us "accentuating the positive" at https://www.facebook.com/compassionateeaters/.

My "eliminating the negative" page is called **The Pinoakesio Diet** and it's an evidence-based critique of one particular Low-Carb Bullshit Artist and, more broadly, it's a science-based refutation of all promoters of high-animal diets, from Atkins, Banting, Cordain, Dukan, Eades, Fallon… to Yudkin and Zone. We're at https://www.facebook.com/The-Pinoakesio-Diet-1661390480774740/.

My LinkedIn profile is at **https://za.linkedin.com/in/rohan-millson-46872126**. On Twitter, I'm **@rohanmillson**.

Other projects with which I'm involved are Greyton Transition Town (GTT), in South Africa, of which I'm currently the secretary, and Greyton Farm Animal Sanctuary, where 16 rescued sheep, 19 pigs, 2 geese, 3 fluffy white chickens and 1 brindled cow (at the time of writing) have me very well-versed in their dietary foibles and sleeping arrangements. Both of these organizations were founded by my extraordinary ex-wife, eternal friend, and Tabularasa Farm partner, Nicola Vernon.

(Our 100-acre farm is off-the-grid, solar-powered, and we built the houses ourselves with the help of eight unconventional builders we trained after spending our honeymoon learning how, from Bill and Athena Steen at the Canelo Project in Arizona; mostly out of straw bales, clay, recycled wood, rock, sand and water. And not in a Fred Flintstone manner either - because their Gaia-friendly materials are within the two-foot-thick clay-plastered walls they're not obvious.)

Greyton Transition Town is the first such sustainable community in Africa. It's our goal to make our surrounding region more resilient in the face of peak oil, climate change and economic instability, and to ameliorate years of racial inequality. Decent housing for all is our #1 priority, followed by humane education in our schools and a host of other projects. If you're interested in seeing more of what we do, or how you can be involved, please visit https://www.greytontransition.co.za.

The **Friends of Greyton Transition Town** congregate at https://www.facebook.com/groups/GTTfriends/. Visitors can stay, inexpensively and comfortably, at GTT's **Greyton EcoLodge** (https://www.facebook.com/ecolodgeatgreyton/), and **Pure Café**

Greyton has a vegan menu and a farmers' market of locally grown produce (https://www.facebook.com/PureCafeGreyton/).

As Nicky and I are both card-carrying vegans, fully aware of the sad pointlessness of eating animals, we've done our best to provide a permanent home for rescued farm animals, who often arrive traumatized or at death's door, or a temporary home for injured or orphaned wild animals, many of whom we've successfully eased out into the wilderness again once they're ready, willing and able to go.

You can find The Greyton Farm Animal Sanctuary at https://www.facebook.com/greytonanimals/. City dwellers, in particular, might enjoy sponsoring one of our beautiful babies as a way of contributing towards the animal liberation movement. Our finances are constrained (shall we say?) and many of our sweeties need parents, so please help out, perhaps even consider adopting one of our babbas from afar [tele-adoption?], if you'd like a simple way to make a big difference in someone else's life. We welcome visitors, and we find that visiting children are often the key that unlocks their parents' hearts (and stomachs).

Devoted animal lovers may like to stay over on the farm, to take part in the pre-dawn feeding of the pigs and geese and other critters. You can find our inexpensive shepherd's hut and barn accommodation on **www.airbnb.com**, under Shepherd's Hut, in Greyton, Western Cape, South Africa.

Nicky and I are both firm believers in community building, so please reach out and make contact with us, especially if your motto is also "For the animals…" Also, despite my best efforts, in a book of this size and ambition there are bound to be errors of commission and omission, of grammar and fact: please let me know my mistakes, and I'll gratefully fix 'em. Naturally, I welcome all *constructive* criticisms and corrections. Thanks. You can send emails to whyanimalsarentfood@gmail.com.

So, that's what my present looks like, and what I have mapped out for the near future… Of course, the Great Unknowable has a whimsical sense of humor and may have entirely different plans for me.

Till later… Be happy, be healthy, be Planter, bye bye.

The End

Parting Snapshot… Saving animals from dire situations can be stressful for people who run animal rescue centers, and 'compassion fatigue' can set in when we're overwhelmed by the nightmares out there. At the Greyton Farm Animal Sanctuary, we've found that just being with the animals is balm to our spirits. Here Iris the pig works her healing magic by letting Nicky give her a full body massage. It's hard to tell who's more contented.

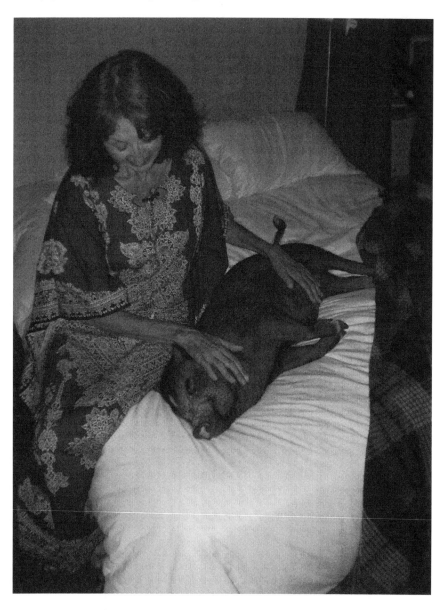

Table of Contents - Book 3

Segue from Book 2 of *Why Animals Aren't Food* (~~Food~~borne Pathogens & Pollutants) iv

Part 4 (Missing in Action) 578

Animal MIAs – Animal Deficiencies 579

  50 Animal Deficiencies That Rule Them Out as Food............................579

    1. Water..579

    2. Chlorophyll..579

    3. Synergistic phytonutrients 582

    4. Nutrient density 582

    5. Plant proteins 583

    5a. Glutamic acid...583

    6. Plant fats..583

    7. Carbohydrates 583

    8. Fiber..584

    9. Phytate ~ phytic acid 585

    10. Gut flora...587

    11. Propionate 588

    12. Lignans 589

    13. Butyrate 590

    14. Minerals..591

    15. Magnesium...591

    16. Calcium...593

    17. Potassium...593

    18. Iodine..594

  Sidebar: A quick rant about the National Nutrient Database............595

    19. Nitrates..597

    20. Phytoestrogens...597

    21. Vitamins 597

    22. Vitamin A...597

23. Folate (Vitamin B9) 598

24. B vitamins (thiamin, riboflavin, niacin, pyridoxine, folate et al).. 598

25. Beta- and the carotenes 599

26. Vitamin C 599

27. Vitamin E 600

28. Vitamin K... 601

29. Ergothioneine 602

30. Salicylic acid.. 603

31. Neurotransmitters, part 1: serotonin.................................. 603

32. Neurotransmitters, part 2: dopamine.................................. 604

33. Neurotransmitters, part 3: adrenaline (epinephrine) 605

Planter mechanisms of optimal health in which Meating is deficient.... 607

34. Antioxidants 607

35. Anti-inflammatories 607

36. Anticarcinogens 608

37. Anti-angiogenesis agents 609

38. Aromatase inhibitors 609

39. DNA repair enzymes 609

40. Epigenetic up- and down-regulators 610

41. IGF-1 Binding Proteins 611

42. Brown fat and the thermogenic effect................................. 611

43. Adiponectin.. 612

44. Leptin and ghrelin 612

45. Mineral absorption enhancers & 'dis-enhancers'................. 613

46. Detoxification enzymes... 613

47. Xenohormesis 613

48. Apoptosis.. 614

49. Natural killer cells... 614

50a. Small intestine immune system activators: Aryl receptors.......... 614

50b. Immune system deactivators in the colon: T$_{regs}$............................ 616

Sidebar: On PREbiotics, PRObiotics and 'RETRObiotics' 618

Stop Press Bonus Meater Deficiencies 619

51. Natural Products That Target Cancer Stem Cells 619

52. Primordial prevention 621

Summary of MIAs 622

Part 5 (Summary): Why Animals Aren't Food   628

When the Cows Come Home to Roost: Consequences of Meating   629

References: Landmarks in medical and nutrition research   631

References to papers on animal and junk components 632

Acrylamide 632

Alpha-gal 632

Ammonia.. 632

Amyloid, cholesterol and Alzheimer's 633

"Animal calories" ~ Brown fat or brown adipose tissue 633

Animal carbohydrates (lactose and galactose)................................ 633

Animal fats (Saturated fats and trans fats) 634

Animal proteins 634

Arachidonic acid... 634

Biogenic amines.. 635

Bones 635

Calcium 635

Carnitine 635

Casein.. 636

Casomorphin 636

Ceramide.. 636

Cholesterol 637

Copper 638

Creatine... 638

Creatinine 638

Diabetogens 639

Diacyl-glycerol 639

Empty calories.. 639

Endotoxins 640

Endocrine disruptors (EDs) 640

Animal Estrogens 641

Feces/Manure/Shit 641

Fish oil 641

Free fatty acids 642

Galactose 642

Gluten ~ Gliadin ~ Wheat protein 642

Harmane 643

Heme iron 643

Heterocyclic amines (PhIP, MeIQx, IQ and IQ4,5b) 644

High Fructose Corn Syrup (HFCS) 644

Homocysteine 644

Hydrogen sulfide 644

IGF-1 (Insulin-like growth factor-1) 645

Junk 645

Lactose 646

LDL cholesterol 646

Methionine 647

Neu5Gc 647

Nitrites 647

Nitrosamines and Nitrosamides/N-nitroso-compounds (NOCs) 648

PhIP 648

Phthalates 649

Phosphorus 649

Polycyclic aromatic hydrocarbons (PAHs) 649

Purines 650

Pus 650

Salt/sodium 650

Steroids ~ sex hormones 651

TMA and TMAO 651

Sidebar: Bacon and eggs - Eggs Bernays? 652

References to papers on "diseases" Meating causes 653

Acne 653

Aggression 653

Aging 654

Alzheimer's "disease" 654

Amputations and Gangrene 655

Angina 655

Asthma 656

Atherosclerosis 656

Birth defects 656

Body odor 658

Breast cancer 658

Breast cancer healed or prevented 659

Cancer 659

Cardiovascular "disease" 661

Cataracts 662

Colon cancer ~ Colorectal cancer 662

Constipation 663

COPD (chronic obstructive pulmonary "disease") 663

Crohn's "disease" 664

Depression 664

Type 1 Diabetes 665

Type 2 Diabetes 665

Gestational diabetes 667

Diabetic retinopathy 667

Diarrhea 667

Disc degeneration & herniation 667

Diverticulosis and Diverticulitis 668

Drug resistance 668

Erectile dysfunction ~ Impotence 669

Fatty liver "disease" 669

Gallstones 670

Glaucoma 670

Gout 671

Guillain-Barré syndrome 671

Heart "disease" (Coronary artery "disease", Cardiac "disease") 671

Hemorrhoids 674

Hiatus hernia 674

Hyperactivity ~ ADHD (Attention Deficit Hyperactivity Disorder) 675

Hypertension 675

Hypertensive retinopathy 675

Iatrogenic deaths 676

Infectious "diseases" 676

Infectobesity 677

Kidney failure 677

Kidney stones 677

Lou Gehrig's "disease" ~ ALS ~ Amyotrophic Lateral Sclerosis 678

Macular degeneration 678

Metabolic syndrome 679

Mood 679

Mortality ~ Death 680

Mucus production 682

Multiple sclerosis 683

Obesity 683

Osteoporosis 684

Parkinson's "disease" 686

Pre-diabetes 686

Premature puberty 687

Prostate cancer 687

Rheumatoid arthritis 688

Sciatica 688

Sexual dysfunction 688

SIDS (Sudden Infant Death Syndrome) ~ Crib Death 689

Stroke (Cerebrovascular "disease") 689

Sudden Cardiac Death.. 689

Ulcerative colitis 690

Urinary tract infections (UTIs) 691

Bacterial vaginosis 691

Yeast infections ~ *Candida*.. 691

References to papers on animal deficiencies.............................. 692

All together now….. 695

A Turd's Eye View of an Animal Meal   696

The Mouth 696

The Esophagus.. 698

The Stomach... 699

The Duodenum.. 701

The Pancreas.. 701

The Liver and Gallbladder 703

Gallstones... 704

Transit time... 705

The enterohepatic circulation of bile...................................... 706

Breast and prostate cancer.. 706

The Small Intestine.. 707

The mesenteric system, or the hepatic portal system.................... 708

Insulin resistance – pre-diabetes - diabetes.............................. 710

The Large Intestine.. 712

The Appendix... 713

Diverticulosis ~ diverticulitis 714

Hemorrhoids (Piles) 714

Other pressure "diseases" 715

Fiber and our gut flora 715

Fatty liver "disease" 719

Kidney failure 719

Auto-immune conditions 719

Atherosclerosis & cardiovascular "disease".................... 720

Leaky gut... 720

Hypertension 721

Dementia.. 722

Cancer... 722

Obesity 723

Lung health 724

Aging... 724

The Meater abyss 724

Death 725

On Silver Bullets & Coffin Nails   728

The Pointlessness of Meating   730

Meating and Earth's Climate   736

The Good News   741

Acknowledgments   743

"What's next?" and "Staying in touch"   745

Table of Contents - Book 3   749

Index to *Why Animals Aren't Food* (complete book)   757

About my next book, *The Low-Carb Bullshit Artists Are Lying Us to Death*   777

Preparing to untie the Gordian Knot.................................... 777

Who, What, Where, When, (How) and Why? (not in that order) 777

The Reality of Nutrition: Animals and Junk Aren't Food 778

The Low-Carb Bullshit Artist Slant on Nutrition 778

Cutting the Low-Carb & Paleo Gordian Knot............................ 779

Why I say most Low-Carb Bullshit Artists are *lying*, not just wrong. 781

Taubesian, adj. overwhelming, as in "Lies of Taubesian proportions". 783

The Meater Hall of Shame ~ Swindlers' List.............................. 790

The Devil's Toolbox - How LCBAs get away with murdering us 792

Outline - *The Low-Carb Bullshit Artists Are Lying Us to Death* 803

Index to *Why Animals Aren't Food* (complete book)

A listing of major topics and personalities

Pages 1-343 as they appear in the complete book are in Book 1,
Pages 344-577 are in Book 2, and
Pages 578 and above are in this book.

(As a bonus, beginning on page 778, this book contains an outline
of the sequel to *Why Animals Aren't Food* called
The Low-Carb Bullshit Artists Are Lying Us to Death.)

2,4,5-TP - 484
Abdominal aortic aneurysm (AAA) - 143
Abdominal fat - 144
Accidents - 144
Acetaldehyde - 484
Acne - 144, 653
Acrylamide - 13, 632
Additives - 484
Adenovirus 36 - 425
ADHD - Attention deficit/hyperactivity disorder - 145
Adrenaline (epinephrine) - 605
Adult onset diabetes - 235
Age-related macular degeneration - 308, 678
AGEs ~ Advanced glycation end-products ~ gerontotoxins - 13
Aggression - 145, 653
Aging - 145, 654
Aldrin/dieldrin - 486
Alkylphenols ~ endocrine disruptors - 487
Allergic responses - 111
Allergies - 151
Alpha-gal - 18, 632
ALS - Amyotrophic lateral sclerosis - 152, 155, 678
Aluminum - 487
Alzheimer's disease - 152, 654
Amides and amines - 18
Ammonia - 19, 489, 632
AMPA - 489

Amputations and gangrene - 288, 655

Amyloid - 19, 633

Amyloidosis - 131

Amyotrophic lateral sclerosis Parkinsonism dementia - 155

Amyotrophic lateral sclerosis (ALS) - 152, 155, 678

Anal fissure - 155

Angina - 155, 655

Animal calories - 20

Animal carbohydrates (lactose and galactose) - 51, 58, 642, 646

Animal estrogens - 43, 641

Animal fats (saturated fats and trans fats) - 21, 634

Animal proteins - 25, 649

Ankylosing spondylitis - 156

Anthrax - 470

Anti-angiogenesis agents - 609

Antibiotics - 490

Antibiotic residues - 510

Antibiotic/antimicrobial resistance - 475, 490

Anticarcinogens - 608

Antidepressants - 491

Antihistamines - 491

Anti-inflammatories - 607

Antioxidants - 607

Antisocial Personality Disorders (ASPDs) - 156

Aphthous ulcers - 156

Apoptosis - 614

Appendix - 713

Arachidonic acid - 29, 634

Aromatase inhibitors - 609

Arsenic - 491

Arteriosclerosis - 81

Arthritis - 156

Artificial flavors - 492

Artificial sweeteners - 493

Aryl receptors - 614

Asbestos - 495

Asthma - 156, 656

Astrovirus - 351

Atheromas - 157

Atherosclerosis - 82, 157,554, 656, 720

Atkins, Dr. Robert ~ Atkins diet - 6, 95, 117-8, 164, 211, 261, 263-4, 564, 705, 752

Atopic dermatitis - 157

Atopic diseases - 157

Attention deficit/hyperactivity disorder (ADHD) - 145

Autism - 158

Auto-immune conditions - 113, 158, 719

Avian leukosis/sarcoma virus - 425

B vitamins (thiamin, riboflavin, niacin, pyridoxine, folate et al) - 598

Bacillus cereus, foodborne - 359

Back pain - 159, 303

Bacteria - 358

Bacterial vaginosis - 158, 690

Bacteriophages - 425

Bacteroides - 106, 200, 588, 589

Bad breath - 160

Banting, William - 237, 261, 263, 752

Barnard, Dr. Neal - 162, 192-3, 196-7, 204, 208-9, 211-212, 227, 241-2, 244, 256, 272, 320, 325, 553, 654, 665, 729, 744-5

Benign prostatic hyperplasia (BPH) - 165

Benzene - 495

Benzo(a)pyrene (B(a)P) - 496

Beta-carboline alkaloids - 497

Beta-carotene - 599

BHA - butylated hydroxyanisole - 497

Bilophila wadsworthia - 106, 108, 200, 528, 588

Biogenic amines - 30, 635

Bio-identical hormones - 497

Birth defects - 160, 656

Bisphosphonates - 497

Bladder infections - 160

Blindness - 160

Blood cancers - 161

Blood clots - 163

BMAA - 465

Body odor - 163, 658

Bone fractures - 163

Bones - 30, 635

Bovine growth hormone ~ bovine somatotropin (rBGH/rBST) - 499

Bovine leukemia virus - 426

Bovine spongiform encephalopathy (BSE) - 169

BPA (Bisphenol A) - 511

Brain disease - 170

Breast and prostate cancer - 674, 703

Breast cancer - 170, 674

Breast cancer healed or prevented - 172, 674

Brown fat ~ brown adipose tissue - 21, 648

Brown fat and the thermogenic effect - 627

Brucella spp. - 370

BSE - Bovine spongiform encephalopathy - 164

Burkitt, Dr. Denis - 91, 94, 274, 276, 584-586, 668, 674

Butcher's warts - 168, 426

Butyrate - 590

Cadaverine - 31

Cadmium - 500

Calcium - 31, 593, 635

Calories - 20, 168

Campbell, Prof. T. Colin - 7, 8, 32, 58, 69, 94, 124-5, 244, 583, 626, 639, 695, 744-5

Campbell, Dr. Thomas - 124-5, 745

Campylobacter spp. - 360

Cancer - 120, 168, 659

Candida - 171, 691

Canker sores - 156

Canthaxanthin - 501

Carbohydrates - 583

Carbon monoxide - 501

Carcinogens - 501, 608

Cardiac arrest - 173

Cardiac disease - 671

Cardiovascular disease - 677

Cardiovascular disease ~ heart disease ~ stroke - 173, 661, 720

Carnitine - 31, 635

Carnosine - 32

Casein - 32, 636

Casomorphin - 32, 636

Cataracts - 175, 662

Celiac disease, gluten sensitivity and wheat allergy - 113

Cellulite - 178

Ceramide - 33, 636

Cerebrovascular disease ~ stroke - 335, 689

Cervical cancer - 179

Cesium - 502

Chan, Dr. Margaret - 277, 389, 446-448

The "Cheese Effect" - 179

Child neglect and child maltreatment - 180

Chlordane - 503

Chlorophyll - 579

Choking - 180

Cholecystokinin - 288

Cholesterol - 33, 504, 637

Choline - 37

Chronic diseases - 180

Chronic dyspepsia (indigestion) - 278

Chronic sequelae of foodborne diseases - 477

Ciguatera - 465

Cirrhosis - 181

Claudication - 93, 182

Clostridial clusters - 102, 105, 617

Clostridium botulinum, foodborne - 366

Clostridium difficile - 432

Clostridium perfringens, foodborne - 366

Colic - 183

Colon cancer ~ colorectal cancer - 182, 662

Constipation - 95, 184, 663

Constipation-type IBS (irritable bowel syndrome) - 185

Contagious pustular dermatitis - 185

Cooking animals at high temperatures - 140

COPD (chronic obstructive pulmonary disease) - 185, 663
Copper - 39, 504, 638
Cordain, Loren, PhD - 6, 653, 752
Coronary artery disease - 671
Cousens, Dr. Gabriel - 256, 272
Creatine - 39, 638
Creatinine - 39, 638
Crib death - 185, 334, 688
Crohn's disease - 186, 664
Cross-contamination - 141
Cyclical mastalgia - 310
Cysteine - 39
Davignon, Dr. Jean - 268, 662, 689
Davis, Brenda, RD - 256, 729, 745
Davis, Dr. William - 6, 256
DDD and DDE - 504
DDT - 505
Death ~ mortality - 680, 725
Deficiencies - 579, 593, 692
Dehydration - 93, 186
Delayed menopause - 187
Dementia - 187
Depression - 191, 664
Deranged gut flora, or microbiome - 98
DES (Diethylstilbestrol) - 506
Detoxification enzymes - 613
Diabetes ~ Diabesity ~ Obesity - 116, 191, 220, 665-7
Diabetes - 116, 191, 220, 665-7
Type 1 diabetes - 665
Type 2 diabetes - 665
Diabetic retinopathy - 273, 667
Diabetogens - 39, 639
Diacetyl - 507
Diacyl-glycerol - 40, 639
Diarrhea - 273, 667
Dieldrin - 486, 507
Diminished penis size - 324

Dioxins and furans - 508

Disc degeneration & herniation - 273, 667

Diverticulosis and diverticulitis - 273, 668, 714

DNA repair enzymes - 609

Domoic acid - 466

Dopamine - 604

Drug residues - 510, 570

Drug resistance - 277, 668

Drugs ~ pharmaceuticals - 510

Drugs other than antibiotics - 512

Dry eye disease - 278

Duodenum - 701

Dyspepsia - 287

E. coli (*Escherichia coli*) - 370

Early menarche/menses - 310

Early-onset diabetes - 220

Eatiology of "diseases" - 143

Eczema - 278

Elective diseases - 278

Embolism - 88, 278

Emphysema - 185, 663

Empty calories - 40, 639

Endocrine disruptors (EDs) - 40, 487, 512, 640

Endometriosis - 279

Endothelial dysfunction - 89

Endotoxemia - 93

Endotoxins - 41, 640

Enterococcus - 436

Enterohepatic circulation of bile - 706

Epigenetic 'up- and down regulators' - 610

Epigenetics - 135

Epilepsy - 281

Erectile dysfunction ~ impotence - 282, 294, 669

Ergothioneine - 602

Escherichia coli (*E. coli*) - 370

Esophagus - 698

Esselstyn, Dr. Caldwell, Jr. - 80, 81, 97, 201, 229, 256, 320, 338, 449, 550, 553, 570, 673, 721, 729, 745

Essential nutrients - 42

Essential tremor - 283

Estradiol - 43

Estrogen - 43, 641

Eye disease - 284

Faecalibacterium prausnitzii - 102-5, 110, 172, 200, 588, 617, 721

Fatty liver disease - 284, 320, 669, 719

Feather meal - 513

Fecal bacteria - 440

Fecal contamination - 49

Feces/manure/shit - 49, 641

Feed additives - 513

Fermentation - 98

Fertilizers - 514

Fiber - 584, 715

Fiber and our gut flora - 715

Fiber deficiency - 94

Fiber-associated nutrient deficiency - 94

Fibromyalgia - 285

Fibrosis - 284

Fish oil - 50, 515, 641

Fish viruses - 426

Flame retardant chemicals - 515

Flatulence - 286

Fluoroquinolones - 516

Folate (Vitamin B$_9$) - 598

Food additives - 484, 516

Food coloring ~ food dyes - 516

Food poisoning - 286

Formaldehyde - 519

Free fatty acids - 50, 642

Fructose - 528, 644

Fuhrman, Dr. Joel - 195, 596, 639, 745

Fungicides - 519

Furans - 508

Gaiacides - 519
Galactose - - 51, 633, 642
Gallbladder - 703
Gallstones - 286, 670, 704
Gangrene and amputations - 288, 655
GERD (Gastro-Esophageal Reflux Disease) - 288
Gerontotoxins - 51
Gestational diabetes - 667
Ghrelin and leptin - 612
Gliadin - 51, 642
Glaucoma - 288, 670
Glutamic acid - 583
Gluten ~ gliadin ~ wheat protein - 51, 642
Glycotoxins - 52
Glyphosate - 519
GMOs - 520
Gout - 289, 670
Greger, Dr. Michael - 1, 13, 18, 19, 29, 35, 42, 50, 51, 59, 66. 70, 74, 84, 89, 94, 95, 116, 117, 129, 130, 143, 146-7, 150, 156, 158, 193, 198, 247-8, 281, 289, 292, 295, 298, 308, 311, 318, 322, 324, 333, 340, 353, 374-5, 378, 413, 423, 432, 444, 455, 480, 483, 488, 506, 525, 526, 532, 545, 549, 563, 582, 586-7, 601, 603-4, 608, 631, 694, 715, 743, 745
Guillain-Barré syndrome - 289, 671
Gut flora - 587
Halitosis - 290
Harmane (Harman) - 52, 522, 643
HAs or HCAs - heterocyclic amines - 55, 524, 644
Hay fever - 290
HDL Cholesterol - 52
Heart disease - 173, 290, 671
Heavy metals - 523
Heiner syndrome - 290
Hemoglobin A1c - 270
Heme iron - 53, 643
Hemorrhoids ~ piles - 291, 674, 714
Hepatic portal system - 708
Hepatitis A virus - 351

Hepatitis E - 426

Herbicides - 524

Heterocyclic amines (HAs or HCAs) - 55, 524, 644

Hexachlorobenzene - 527

HFCS – High fructose corn syrup - 528, 644

Hiatus hernia - 291, 674

High blood pressure - 291

High fructose corn syrup (HFCS) - 528, 644

Himsworth, Dr. HP - 243, 256

Homocysteine - 55, 644

Hormonal dysfunction - 291

Hormones - 43

Human papilloma virus (HPV) - 427

Hydrogen sulfide (H_2S) - 56, 528, 644

Hyman, Dr. Mark - 6, 665

Hyperactivity ~ ADHD - 292, 675

Hypercholesterolemia - 81

Hyper-filtration and protein leakage - 86

Hyperlipidemia - 82

Hypertension - 292, 675, 721

Hypertensive retinopathy - 292, 675

Hypoperfusion - 78

Hypospadias - 293

Hypoxia and Anoxia - 78

Iatrogenic deaths - 293, 676

IBDs (Inflammatory bowel diseases) - 297

IBS (Irritable bowel syndrome) - 298

IGF-1 (Insulin-like growth factor-1) - 57, 645

IGF-1 binding proteins (IBPs) - 611

Immune and auto-immune responses - 111

Immune system deactivators in the colon: T_{regs} - 616

Impotence - 294, 669

Inadequate bowel movements - 164

Indigestion ~ chronic dyspepsia - 278

Industrial pollutants/toxins - 528

Infarction - 88, 319

Infectious diseases - 294, 676

Infectobesity - 294, 677
Infertility - 295
Inflammation - 77
Inflammatory bowel diseases (IBDs) - 297
Insecticides - 529
Insulin resistance - 297
Insulin resistance – pre-diabetes - diabetes - 782
Insulin-like growth factor-1 - 57, 645
Intermittent claudication - 93, 182
Iodine - 594
IQ and IQ4,5b - 57, 644
Iron - 53, 529, 643
Irritable bowel syndrome (IBS) - 298
Ischemia - 78
Jaundice - 298
Jenkins, Dr. David J - 242, 252-4, 268, 662, 665, 673-4, 689
Joy, Melanie, PhD - 745, 748
Junk - 57, 645
Kempner, Dr. Walter - 256, 327, 675, 729
Keriorrhea - 466
Ketosis - 117
Kidney failure - 299, 677, 719
Kidney stones - 301, 677
Klaper, Dr. Michael - 31, 256, 700, 707, 746
Lactescence - 79
Lactose - 58, 633, 646
Large intestine - 712
Lauric acid - 58
LDL cholesterol - 59, 646
Lead - 530
Leaky gut - 111, 720
Leptin and ghrelin - 612
Leucine - 59
Leukemias - 302
Lignans - 589
Lindane - 530
Lipoproteins - 59

Listeria monocytogenes - 378
Liver and gallbladder - 703
Liver disease - 284, 303, 320, 669, 719
Longevity - 303
Lou Gehrig's disease ~ ALS - 303, 678
Lower back pain - 159, 303
Lower IQ - 297
Lower sperm counts & poor semen quality - 334
Lung health - 724
Lupus erythematosus - 304
Lymphomas - 308
Macular degeneration - 308, 678
Magnesium - 591
Marek's disease virus - 427
Mastalgia - 310
McDougall, Dr. John - 1, 17, 47, 52, 97, 126, 156, 196, 216, 224, 244, 256,
    272, 334, 423, 526, 570, 683, 688, 729, 744, 746
Meat - 59
Meat glue - 531
Mechanically separated meat - 59
MeIQx - 60, 644
Early menarche/menses - 310
Delayed menopause - 187
Mental health - 310
Mercola, Dr. Joseph - 555-558, 608
Mercury - 532
Mesenteric system - 708
Metabolic acidosis - 86
Metabolic syndrome - 312, 679
Metastatic calcification - 86
Methionine - 60, 647
MGUS - 315
Microalbuminuria - 315
Microparticles - 534
Milk apnea - 315
Mills, Dr. Milton - 626, 697
Mineral absorption enhancers & 'dis-enhancers' - 613

Minerals - 591
Mirex (Dechlorane) - 532
Miscellany: skin, cartilage, tendons - 60
Molecular mimicry - 315
Monsanto - 280, 281, 448, 489, 519-20, 540, 551, 639, 733
Mood - 315, 679
Mortality ~ death - 316, 484, 680, 725
Mouth - 696
MRSA (Methicillin- (or multi-drug-) resistant *Staphylococcus aureus*) - 441
Mucus production - 317, 682
Multiple myeloma - 317
Multiple sclerosis - 318, 682
Muscle wasting - 82, 86, 301, 613
Muscular atony - 319
Mutagens - 534
Mycobacterium bovis - 382
Myocardial infarction - 319
Myoglobin - 61
Myristic acid - 61
Nanoparticles - 534
National Nutrient Database - 595
Natural killer cells - 614
Natural Products that target cancer stem cells - 619-621
Nematodes (roundworms) - 410, 455
Neonicotinoids - 535
Neu5Gc - 62, 647
Neurotoxins - 535
Nitrates - 597
Nitrites - 62, 535, 647
Nitrosamines and Nitrosamides - 63, 537, 648
N-nitroso-compounds (NOCs) - 61, 65, 648
Noakes, Prof. Tim - 6, 109-110, 556, 626, 752
Nonalcoholic fatty liver disease - 320
Non-Hodgkin's lymphoma - 321
Norovirus - 352
Nutrient density - 582
Nutrigenomics - 167

www.nutritionfacts.org - 13, 18, 19, 29, 30, 35, 42, 51, 70, 71, 81, 84, 89, 104, 107, 130, 148, 151, 193, 198, 203, 247, 249, 252, 281, 288, 289, 292, 297, 298, 308, 311, 318, 322, 324, 333, 339, 341, 353, 378, 420, 432, 444, 455, 480, 483, 488, 506, 526, 545, 549, 582, 586, 603, 604, 605, 608, 631, 716, 743

Obesity ~ diabesity ~ diabetes - 116

Obesity - 191, 321, 683, 723

Obesogens - 64, 537

Octachlorostyrene - 538

Omega-3 fatty acids - 64

Omega-6 fatty acids - 66

Oncogenic, or cancer-causing, viruses - 427

Oral lichen planus - 321

Organochlorines - 538

Organophosphates - 539

Organotins - 539

Ornish, Dr. Dean - 7, 36, 124, 137, 149, 157, 170, 174, 181, 256, 283, 386, 553, 558, 570, 610, 654, 665, 672-3, 687, 729, 743-4, 746

Osteoarthritis - 321

Osteoporosis - 322, 684

Ovarian cancer - 323

Oxidation ~ oxidative stress - 78

PAHs - polycyclic aromatic hydrocarbons - 68, 539, 548, 649

Painter, Dr. Neil S - 274, 668

Palmitic acid - 67

Pancreas - 701

Pancreatic cancer - 323

Paralysis - 324

Parasites - 399, 452, 455

Parkinson's disease - 324, 685

PBDEs - Polybrominated diphenylethers - 540

PBTs - Persistent, bioaccumulative, and toxic pollutants - 542

PCBs - Polychlorinated biphenyls - 540, 547

PCRM - Physicians Committee for Responsible Medicine - 162, 211, 565, 646, 709, 730, 744

Peptic ulcer - 324

Perfluorochemicals - 541

Peripheral artery disease - 325
Peripheral neuropathy - 133
Perlmutter, Dr. David - 6, 526, 625
Persistent, bioaccumulative, and toxic (PBT) pollutants - 542
Persistent organic pollutants (POPs) - 543
Pesticides - 544
PhIP - 67, 644, 648
Phosphate additives - 544
Phosphorus - 67, 649
Phthalates - 545, 649
Phytate ~ phytic acid - 585
Phytoestrogens - 597
Pink slime - 68, 546
Piles ~ hemorrhoids - 291, 674, 714
PITS - Perpetration-induced traumatic stress - 325
Plant fats - 583
Plant proteins - 583
Platelet hyperreactivity - 81
Polonium - 547
Polybrominated diphenylethers (PBDEs) - 540
Polycarbonate plastic - 547
Polychlorinated biphenyls (PCBs) - 540, 547
Polychlorinated naphthalenes (PCNs) - 548
Polycyclic aromatic hydrocarbons (PAHs) - 68, 539, 548, 649
Polyps - 325
POPs - Persistent organic pollutants - 543
Porcine endogenous retroviruses - 430
Potassium - 593
Potassium sorbate - 549
Poultry viruses - 430
Pre-diabetes - 326, 686, 710
Pre-eclampsia - 326
Pre-hypertension - 326
Premature puberty - 327, 686
Preservatives - 550
Pressure diseases - 327, 715
Prevotella - 106, 200-1, 588

Primordial prevention - 621

Prion disease - 327

Prions - 462

Pritikin, Nathan - 91-2, 256, 729

Prolactin - 68

Propionate - 588

Prostate cancer - 327, 687, 706

Proteins - 25, 583, 634

Proteus mirabilis - 440

Protozoa - 399

Psoriasis - 328

Psychopathy and sociopathy - 330

Psyllium husks - 550

Purge - 68

Purines - 69, 650

Pus - 69, 650

Putrefaction - 97

Putrescine - 70

Rabies - 430

Ractopamine - 551

Reticuloendotheliosis virus - 431

Rheumatoid arthritis - 332, 687

Roberts, Dr. William C. - 656

Rotavirus - 354

Rouleau(x) formation - 79

Roundup® - 551

Roundworms (nematodes) - 410, 455

Salicylic acid - 603

Salmonella enterica serotype Typhi - 382

Salmonella spp., nontyphoidal - 382

Salt/sodium - 70, 551, 650

Sapovirus - 355

Sarcoidosis - 333

Saturated fats - 70, 634

SCD - Sudden cardiac death - 336, 689

Sciatica - 333, 688

Sclerosis - 81

Scombroid poisoning - 467

Scurvy - 333

Seizures - 333

Semen quality - 334

Serotonin - 603

Sex hormones ~ steroid hormones - 43, 651

Sexual dysfunction - 333, 688

Shaken baby syndrome - 183

Shaper, Dr. AG - 274, 672

Shearer, Mary-Ann and Mark - 744

Shellfish poisoning - 467

Shigella spp. - 388

SIDS - Sudden infant death syndrome - Crib death - 185, 338, 688

Sludging of the blood ~ lactescence - 79

Small intestine - 707

Small intestine immune system activators: Aryl receptors - 614

Small stool size - 334

Sociopathy - 334

Sodium benzoate - 552

Sodium/salt - 70, 551, 650

Spence, Dr. JD - 268, 646, 662, 689

Sperm counts - 334

Spermidine - 71

Spermine - 71

Spina bifida - 334

Staphylococcus aureus & MRSA (Methicillin-resistant *Staphylococcus aureus*) - 441

Statins - 552

Stearic acid - 71

Stenosis - 87

Steroid hormones ~ sex hormones - 43, 651

Stomach - 699

Straining at stool - 334

Streptococcus - 389

Streptococcus spp. Group A, foodborne - 389

Stroke (cerebrovascular disease) - 346, 705

Sudden cardiac death (SCD) - 336, 689

Sudden infant death syndrome (SIDS) - Crib death - 185, 338, 688

Sugar - 554

Sugar and cancer; sugar and atherosclerosis - 554

Suicide - 338

Sulfites - 573

Sulfur - 71

Sulfur dioxide (SO$_2$) - 560

Sulfur-containing amino acids - 72

Supplements - 561, 564

Surgery, chemotherapy and radiation - 338

Swank, Dr. Roy Laver - 158, 682-3, 729

Sweeney, Dr. J. Shirley - 256

Swine flu - 470

Synergistic phytonutrients - 582

Synthetic growth hormones - 522

Tapeworms - 457

Taubes, Gary - 6, 218, 265, 557, 610

Taurine - 72

Teicholz, Nina - 6, 557, 610

Teratogens - 564

Testicular cancer - 339

Tetrahydroisoquinoline - 565

Tetrodotoxin - 468

Thrombosis - 88

Thrush - 171

Titanium dioxide - 565

TMA and TMAO - 72, 651

Tobacco smoke - 565, 574

Toxaphene - 566

Toxemia - 111

Trans fats - 21, 72, 567, 634

Transglutaminase - 569

Transit time - 339, 705

T$_{regs}$ - regulatory T-cells - 616

Trichinella - 410

Triclosan and Triclocarban - 56

Triglycerides - 72

Trowell, Dr. Hugh - 274, 276, 584

TSEs - Transmissible spongiform encephalopathies - 462

Tuberculosis (TB) - 132

Tuttle, Will, PhD - iii - iv, 120, 744, 746

Twin births - 339

Type 1 Diabetes - 191, 220, 665

Type 2 Diabetes - 191, 220, 665, 710

Tyramine - 179

Ulcerative colitis - 339, 690

Uric acid - 73

Urinary tract infections (UTIs) - 340, 690

Uterine cancer - 341

Vaginosis - 159, 690

Varicose veins - 341

Vegetable oils - 569

Venous thromboses - 341

Veterinary drug residues - 570

Vibrio cholerae, toxigenic - 390

Vibrio parahaemolyticus - 394

Vibrio spp., other - 394

Vibrio vulnificus, the "flesh-eating bacterium" - 391

Vinclozolin - 570

Viruses - 351-356, 425-431

Vitamin A - 597

B vitamins (thiamin, riboflavin, niacin, pyridoxine, folate et al) - 598

Vitamin B_{12} - 571

Vitamin C - 599

Vitamin D - 33, 219, 274, 561, 581, 593, 620, 664

Vitamin E - 600

Vitamin K - 601

Vitamins - 571, 597

VLDL - 74

Walsh, Bryan - 557, 610

Warfarin - 572

Wart viruses - 431

Water - 579

Water 'deficiency' ~ dehydration - 93, 186

Weight management - 219

Wheat protein ~ gluten ~ gliadin - 51, 113, 642

Wheeze - 341

Whey - 74

Williams, Dr. Kim - 175

Wrinkles - 341

Xeno-autoantibodies - 74

Xenoestrogens - 75, 573

Xenohormesis - 613

Yeast infections ~ Candida - 171, 341, 691

Yersinia enterocolitica - 395

Zeranol - 576

Zinc - 576

Zoönotic diseases - 342, 469

Zugzwang - 75

~

About my next book,
The Low-Carb Bullshit Artists Are Lying Us to Death

Preparing to untie the Gordian Knot

Legend has it that before Alexander could set off eastwards from Macedonia to Conquer The World (and so become Alexander the Great), he had to perform a task that had stymied all-comers before him. He had to undo a huge and hugely complicated knot tied by King Gordius of Phrygia. Alexander's elegant solution was to whip out his sword and slice the thing in two. After some preamble, I'm going to *remind* you how to emulate Alexander and slice through the low-carb (high-animal) Gordian knot.

Who, What, Where, When, (How) and Why? (not in that order)

Because we know *Why Animals Aren't Food*, and because the evidence for this has become overwhelming since 1990*, the Low-Carb Bullshit Artists and their Paleo sidekicks (and the believers in "all things in moderation"), acting in the present to protect vested interests in academia and the medical, drug, "food" and other industries, are forced to tell untruths and outright lies about nutrition science to perpetuate the deadly and profitable myth that we can eat animals without suffering severe health consequences.

I've identified a Devil's Toolbox of 50 Lying Techniques which appear over and over in nasty low-carb and paleo diet books; in the curricula of medical and dietetic and veterinary schools; in prestigious medical journals; on the websites of initialized, disease-combatting, telethon-running non-profit organizations; in the advice given by government health, agriculture, food and drug departments; and, especially, in the US's 5-yearly dietary guidelines, all of which continue to promote the practice of eating animals, despite all the best evidence showing how dangerous and how deadly it is.

With reference to 1990*, above, I choose 1990 as the year since which we've known for sure that animals aren't food, because that's the year Dean Ornish and his fellow researchers demonstrated conclusively that banishing animals from our diet banishes our #1 cause of death. What more should we need to know about how to eat?

Ornish D, Brown SE, Scherwitz LW, Billings JH, Armstrong WT, Ports TA, McLanahan SM, Kirkeeide RL, Brand RJ, Gould KL. Can lifestyle changes reverse coronary heart disease? The Lifestyle Heart Trial. *Lancet*. 1990 Jul 21;336(8708):129-33. [The medical landmark of landmarks.]

The Reality of Nutrition: Animals and Junk Aren't Food

When we eat, we eat combinations of three things - processed animals, processed plants and whole plants. These three things contain nutrients and other substances that aren't nutrients.

Whole, veganically-grown plants contain nothing but nutrients, and eating them brings nothing but good health - they qualify as food.

(In *Why Animals Aren't Food* I dealt with 2 minor drawbacks to Planting - vitamin B_{12}, and celiac disease & wheat/gluten/gliadin sensitivities.)

Processed things - whether of plant or animal origin - contain all sorts of unavoidable substances that aren't good for us, either innate (such as arachidonic acid, amyloid, Neu5Gc, PhIP and dozens of others I described in *Why Animals Aren't Food*) or externally supplied (such as heavy metals, PCBs, dioxins, DDT, preservatives and hundreds of others). The animals we eat also contain almost all the pathogens that kill tens of thousands of us each year. Processed plants (junk) and animals are both notoriously energy-dense and nutrient-deficient. Junking and Meating cause nothing but bad health outcomes. Junk and animals are therefore not food.

Good nutritionists focus on Meating, Junking and Planting (without necessarily thinking in those terms) to work out what effects the food "package deal" has on the human body in the present, and right where most of us live, in the cities of industrializing nations. When done 'wholistically,' good nutrition science today shows with 100% certainty that eating animals is our real #1 cause of death, with Junking and smoking vying for #2.

The Low-Carb Bullshit Artist Slant on Nutrition

Because the "package deal" of animals-as-food is obviously such a nutrition disaster zone when considered holistically, Meaters try to fool the gullible into Meating (or try to give the Meaters who "love" animals too much to give them up a rationale for carrying on eating them) by getting us to focus on irrelevances and distractions such as :

- Sugar as the supposed (& easily disproven) sole cause of disease,
- Reductionism, especially about cholesterol and vitamin B_{12},
- Weight loss,
- Human evolution, and
- Outlier populations such as the Inuit and the Maasai.

While I only have space and time to skim over each of these LCBA diversions in this introduction to *The Low-Carb Bullshit Artists Are Lying Us to Death*, I go into them in some detail in the book itself.

Cutting the Low-Carb & Paleo Gordian Knot

I believe I provided the sword that cuts the high-animal diet Gordian knot when I wrote *Why Animals Aren't Food.* In it I described more than 200 instances of animal components, pathogens, pollutants and deficiencies which are harmful to us, and I described the mechanisms whereby these substances and parasites harm and kill us, thus proving that animals aren't food. Junk has similar effects and also isn't food. Only whole plants qualify.

So when a Low-Carb Bullshit Artist says we should eat animals to get some nutrient or other... or if a paleo-pest tells us we ate animals 60 million years ago, therefore we should eat animals today... or if some total twit tells us we should eat animals because of our blood type... or if a reasonable-sounding individual tells us we should show moderation in all things, and veganism is immoderate... or if a stupid twit or a dishonest tw*t confuses cause for effect and tells us that sugar causes cancer, rather than that low-oxygen conditions (caused by atherosclerosis, caused by cholesterol) cause cancer cells to ferment sugar anaerobically... or if we want to understand why so many of the low-carb and paleo hucksters are fat and ill, while all my Planter role models are slender and healthy (and some of them are aging rather splendidly)... it's easy to cut the high-animal Gordian knot...

Just say: "Animals aren't food."

When we *know* animals aren't food, it doesn't matter what rationale Low-Carbers and other Meat marketers give us for buying their bloody wares. Their first principle is wrong; their *a priori* assumption. When they say: "Buy this food because it..." we cut them off right there and say: "You can skip the "because" rigmarole, because it ain't food." Logic applies- if A, then B... but Meating's not-A, therefore don't try to foist B on me.

They say: "Buy this airplane because..." and we interject: "Stop (in the name of love) right there. Having wings and wheels don't make it a plane - that sucker can't fly." Just because we eat it, doesn't make it food.

That's how easy it is to cut the Gordian knot of Low-Carb Bullshit Artistry.

It doesn't matter if there's stuff that might be good for us in the animal package when the rest of the package sickens and kills us.

It doesn't matter what we ate tens or hundreds or thousands of thousands of years ago when animals aren't food *today*, and eating them *today* kills us before our time, today.

It doesn't matter what blood group we are. The animals don't differentiate between blood types - not being food, they kill all of us, from A to O.

It doesn't matter how much we prize the concept of moderation when eating moderately leads to being only moderately healthy and living a moderately long life. I prefer to be immoderately, exuberantly healthy.

And it doesn't matter to Planters how harmful processed sugar is, because we don't eat that either - it's junk, not food. But when we eat mass quantities of sugar-packed whole plants - an extremely high whole-carb, no-animal diet - then we enjoy peak health and longevity.

There it is: we can slice through all the arguments of the Low-Carb Bullshit Artists and all the other proponents of high-animal eating when we carry the simple, yet keen-edged Planter nutrition sword, sharper than Occam's razor (or a serpent's tooth), which is the absolute knowledge that…

Animals aren't food.

I have more to say about all this in both *Why Animals Aren't Food* and *The Low-Carb Bullshit Artists Are Lying Us to Death*. In the remainder of this intro to the latter book, I'm going to sprint through the following three topics, before closing with a chapter-level book outline:

- **Why I know the Low-Carbers are lying, not just mistaken**. That's easy to show - "by their deeds shall you know them." I dig a couple of spadefuls of shit from the steaming pile in the first two pages of Chapter 1 of Lying Low-Carb Snake #1, Gary Taubes's *Good Calories, Bad Calories*, and present them as an archetype of deviousness.
- In **The Meater Hall of Shame**, I list without discussing them the writers and writings I'll be putting under the scope of my bullshit-o-meter in *Bullshit Artists*. Not all of them are low-carbers; not all of them are liars; they're all Meaters who're wrong about animals-as-food.
- In **The Devil's Toolbox**, I list and briefly describe scores of tools for lying whose handles the Low-Carb and Paleo Bullshit Artists have worn smooth by using them so often. In the book I flesh out this section with plenty of examples, naming names.

Okay. Here goes…

But first, a quick note on my disrespectful tone…

I'm not someone who calls a spade a "portable excavation implement." When I think that Tim Noakes, for example, is being a lying, conniving weasel, as I often do, I'll call him a lying, conniving weasel, even if in so doing I defame all weasels everywhere. I'll apologize to the next one I meet.

If you think I'm launching unfair *ad hominem* or *ad feminam* attacks against the Low-Carb Bullshit Artists, calling them nasty names in order to make my point, then think again. This isn't so. I call them names because they're dangerous and they piss me off. If you bear with me, you'll soon see that I'm calling these nasty people nasty names because their behavior is so scurrilous, and the damage they do us and our Earth so outrageous.

I've *earned* the right to call the Low-Carb Bullshit Artists nasty names, having spent years in their odious company, feeling psychically polluted by their complete lack of ethics and their complete lack of empathy, bewildered by the warm reception they receive from their doting followers, and powerless to save now-dead loved ones from their clutches.

Like Howard Beale, Peter Finch's character in *Network*, "I'm mad as hell and I'm not going to take it any more."

Hence this invective-packed book, in which I ask you: What's to respect?

Why I say most Low-Carb Bullshit Artists are *lying*, not just wrong
Because you've read *Why Animals Aren't Food*, you're more than halfway to knowing that *The Low-Carb Bullshit Artists Are Lying Us to Death*.

We don't yet know for sure that they're *lying*, these proponents of high-animal diets. We do know, with absolute certainty, hundreds of reasons why they're wrong. (And if amateurs like us know the enormous body of science that proves this, how can the low-carb pros not know? Are they dense?)

Once we understand the damage they cause us, we'd have to be stupid, ignorant, deluded or insane to advise others to eat animals. Is there an option I've left out? Yes. Evil, of an active and a "just following orders" kind, the second of which Hannah Arendt referred to in her *Eichmann in Jerusalem* as "the banality of evil" - the inertia or momentum of the Meater status quo.

Stupid people may promote Meating because they lack the mental capacity to understand the science.

Ignorant people, likewise, because, smart or dumb, they haven't yet learned the science.

Deluded people, ditto, because they've been misinformed, enculturated, edumacated, propagandized, public relationed, advertised, dietary guidelined and low-carb (and paleo) bullshitted into believing animals are food.

Crazy people, too, because they lack a coherent attachment to reality, so their judgment is impaired.

But evil people… the psychopaths among nutrition writers… these people know they're wrong about animals-as-food, and yet they persist with their maniacal Meater message.

In *The Low-Carb Bullshit Artists Are Lying Us to Death* I'll show why I think many writers of low-carb, paleo and other high-animal weight loss books aren't just wrong; they know they're wrong and, because the evidence against Meating is so Everest-like, they have to tell lies to maintain the illusion of animals-as-food. Sloppy science can only take them so far.

The knowledge that animals aren't food has entered and is transforming mainstream palliative medicine. Preventive Planting and its application in lifestyle medicine are upsetting the drug-fuelled Meater medical establishment, which is resisting change, tooth and claw. We see this most clearly in the refusal by medical boards and medical schools to mandate nutrition education for doctors. As a result, today's medical practitioners are being deprived of their most powerful healing tool - plants-only nutrition. If it doesn't change soon, conventional medicine runs the risk of becoming like conventional agriculture… an outdated liability.

As Dr. Kim Williams, the director of the American Council of Cardiology, says: "There are two kinds of cardiologists: vegans, and those who haven't read the data." Think about that. Not a word about cholesterol: Dr. Williams says *eating animals kills our hearts*. We need to think wholistically, in terms of whole classes of 'foods,' not single substances.

IARC (the International Agency for Research on Cancer), a unit of the World Health Organization, published a press release on 26 October 2015 called "Carcinogenicity of consumption of red and processed meat." It says "processed meats" such as deli meats and jerky are Group 1 carcinogens, the same cancer-causing level as smoking and asbestos. "Red meat" is in Group 2 and is implicated in pancreatic, colorectal and prostate cancer.

[*Lancet Oncol* S1470-2045(15)00444-1 (http://dx.doi.org/10.1016/)]

Frankly, real scientists have known for decades about the toxicity of all animals, not just processed or red meat, but it's great that large and influential health organizations are standing up and confirming the science.

How then do the Low-Carb Bullshit Artists manage to sidestep the science, a Marianas Trench of which I presented in *Why Animals Aren't Food* to show that Meating is our #1 killer? Surely it's a drawback in a diet that it causes heart disease and cancer and shortens our lives? I've long wanted to know whether the low-carbers are stupid, ignorant, deluded, insane or evil.

To help solve that riddle, let me introduce you to PlantPositive. The website of the pseudonymous researcher known as PlantPositive (found at http://www.plantpositive.com/) provides by far the most thorough review of low-carbism and paleo diets. His vivisection of the Low-Carb Bullshit Artists and their Paleo playmates is compelling, well-referenced and extremely entertaining (for those not being skewered and roasted).

Now, with his help, to give you an idea of how rotten-to-the-core Low-Carbism is, let's take a look at how the modern Low-Carb Bullshit Artist-in-Chief operates. The following section is about ex-journalist Gary Taubes.

Taubesian, adj. overwhelming, as in "Lies of Taubesian proportions"

I chose Taubes as an exemplar of the Low-Carb Bullshit Artists for several reasons. He's the vector of the latest outbreak of the low-carb plague that seems to lie dormant for a generation and then break out again with increased virulence, killing thousands before getting stamped out again. This time is different. Big money is involved, and the infection has spread even into the *British Medical Journal,* which has published some of Taubes's scribblings. Another reason is that Taubes used to be a respected science writer and many unsuspecting dupes have trusted him, cribbing and repeating many of his nutrition lies. He's probably the most influential of the high-animal bullshitters.

It's instructive to read the drivel he ladles out in Chapter 1 of his *Good Calories, Bad Calories* (2007) after watching PlantPositive's video on the subject, to see just what a prodigious liar Gary Taubes is.

[See: "The Journalist Gary Taubes 2: A Parajournalism Paradox" at www.plantpositive.com.]

Chapter 1 is called "The Eisenhower Paradox." In it Taubes would like us
to empathize with An American Hero who ate a (supposedly) heart-healthy,
(supposedly) low-fat, (supposedly) low-cholesterol diet but who somehow
still died of a heart attack.

Absolute bollocks. None of these supposed things is true.

Taubes's ulterior motive for fabricating a cock-and-bull story about ex-
president Dwight Eisenhower's diet and his heart disease is to leave us with
the false impression that a true low-fat, low-cholesterol diet isn't heart-
protective. Taubes sets up a phony "low-fat, low-cholesterol" diet as a
"straw man," easy to knock down. His goal with this concocted anecdote
about Ike is to discredit an early proponent of the cholesterol theory, the
great Ancel Keys, and thereby to discredit the cholesterol theory itself, so
that we may feel a false sense of safety when eating animals.

(To understand how scabrous this is, keep in mind that Taubes knows that
Dean Ornish proved without a doubt in 1990 that a no-animal diet reverses
coronary heart disease. Cholesterol is just one of dozens of animal
components that kill us. Got animals? Got disease.)

Taubes wants to fool us into believing that Eisenhower was eating a low-fat,
low-cholesterol diet, and here's how he describes Eisenhower's first heart
attack in the first paragraph of the first chapter of *Good Calories, Bad Calories*,
on page 3:

"It may have started on Friday, September 23, 1955. Eisenhower had spent
that morning playing golf and lunched on **a hamburger with onions**, [all
emphases added] which gave him what appeared to be indigestion."

Hmm, I guess it was a low-fat, low-cholesterol, heart-healthy hamburger.

Unmentioned by Taubes, but not difficult to find in this paper, cited by
PlantPositive - Anastasia Kucharski. Medical management of political
patients: the case of Dwight D. Eisenhower. *Perspect Biol Med*. 1978
Autumn;22(1):115-26 - here's what Eisenhower had eaten for breakfast on
the day of his first heart attack, before lunching on a hamburger and
(probably fried) onions: "**sausage, bacon, mush, and hot cakes**."

Must have been low-fat bacon. And tofurkey sausage. (Faux turkey?) Why
would Taubes not mention such heart-healthy fare?

Here's what Taubes *chose to include* in his book concerning Eisenhower's
health and habits:

"We know that he had no family history of heart disease, and **no obvious risk factors** after he quit smoking in 1949. He exercised regularly; his weight remained close to the 172 pounds considered optimal for his height. His blood pressure was only occasionally elevated. His cholesterol was below normal: his last measurement before the attack, according to George Mann... was 165 mg/dl (milligrams/deciliter), a level that heart-disease specialists today consider safe."

I devote several pages in *The Low-Carb Bullshit Artists Are Lying Us to Death* to decontaminating all the crap Taubes packed into just this one paragraph. (It takes a lot of work to clean up after these people.) Here's some of what Mr. Devious *chose to exclude* about Eisenhower's habits and health:

- Eisenhower had Crohn's disease, an inflammatory bowel condition, for the last 46 years of his life,
- He had three operations to remove intestinal obstructions,
- He developed type 2 diabetes later in life,
- After his death [!], his autopsy showed he had a pheochromocytoma, a tumor on one of his adrenal glands,
- Although Taubes does tell us Ike had quit smoking cigarettes six years earlier, he doesn't mention he'd been a heavy smoker, going through 3 to 4 packs a day,
- He'd also been a heavy coffee drinker, drinking up to 15 cups a day, and
- He ate "high-grade protein with each meal," meaning lots of animals, including "steak for breakfast" and "fried chicken."

The book that Taubes quotes from and suppresses in such unequal measure is Clarence Lasby's *Eisenhower's Heart Attack: How Ike Beat Heart Disease and Held on to the Presidency* (University Press of Kansas, 1997).

Now tell me, after seeing what's in Lasby's book, which Taubes lists in his bibliography, so I assume he's read it: if you were trying to tell someone a great truth, would you tell them as many lies of omission as Taubes just did? And we've only finished the first page of chapter 1, God help us.

Here are the dietary changes Ike made, according to Taubes [*GCBC* p. 4]:

"After his heart attack, **Eisenhower dieted religiously** and had his cholesterol measured ten times a year. **He ate little fat and less cholesterol**; his meals were cooked in either **soybean oil** or **a newly**

developed polyunsaturated margarine, which appeared on the market in 1958 as a **nutritional palliative for high cholesterol**."

Keep in mind that Caldwell Esselstyn, one of today's foremost heart healers, has a mantra for healing hearts. It's "No oil!" Does anyone besides Taubes think that Eisenhower is now eating the epitome of a true low-fat, low-cholesterol, heart-healthy diet? If you do, I have a bridge to sell you. The man was eating junk, not food.

Where's Taubes going with this crapola? Enter the villain… the foremost nutrition researcher of Ike's day, Ancel Keys.

"Eisenhower's cholesterol hit 259 just six days after University of Minnesota physiologist Ancel Keys made the cover of *Time* magazine [on 13 January 1961], **championing precisely the kind of supposedly heart-healthy diet on which Eisenhower had been losing his battle with cholesterol for five years**. It was two weeks later that the American Heart Association - prompted by Keys's force of will [AHA wusses!] - published its first official endorsement of low-fat, low-cholesterol diets as a means to prevent heart disease."

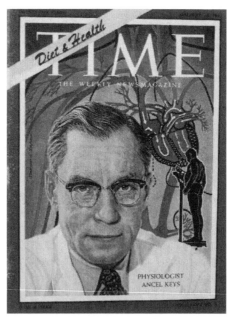

Now, to give Taubes his due: Keys did say that vegetable oils are better for us than animal fats. But what else did Keys say about how we should be eating to stay well? In fact, who was Ancel Keys?

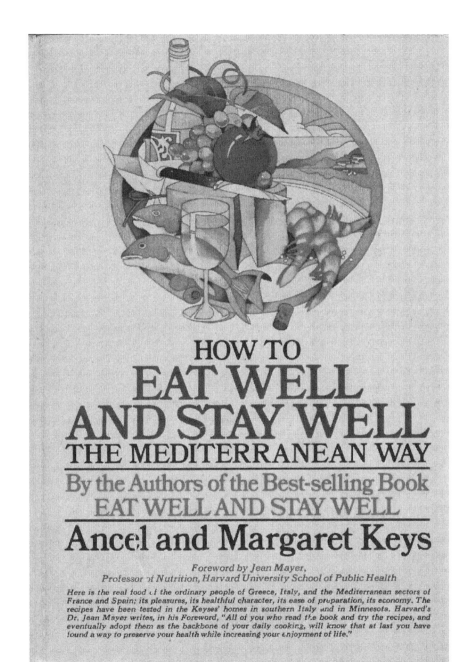

Ancel & Margaret Keys. *Eat Well and Stay Well The Mediterranean Way* (1963)

Among half a dozen major scientific achievements in his career, any one of which would have been the jewel in another scientist's crown, Keys was the 'inventor' of the Mediterranean diet. I devote a chapter of *The Low-Carb Bullshit Artists* to restoring this great man's reputation, which liars like Taubes and his many copycats have stolen from him since his death.

Take a look at the cover of Ancel and Margaret Keys' book, *Eat Well and Stay Well The Mediterranean Way*, published in January 1963, to get some idea of Keys' thinking about nutrition in the early 1960s.

What do we see? Fishes, crustaceans like langoustines or prawns, wine, cheese, olive oil, olives, tomatoes and grapes. Fresh, whole fruits and vegetables. And animals, to be sure - almost no one back then knew just how detrimental to our health the eating of animals is, and the cholesterol theory was still in its infancy. Keys certainly didn't propose a vegan diet.

So, which of the foods Ancel Keys recommended in his book was Eisenhower eating while he "dieted religiously," as Taubes puts it? How many times does Taubes mention grapes or apples or tomatoes or broccoli or spinach in connection with Eisenhower? Heck, even fishes or cheese or wine, unhealthy as they are? Yes, you're right if your answer is zero. When it came to plants, nothing but the best mush, deep-fried-in-Brylcreem or some such oleaginous "nutritional palliative" junk would do for Dwight David.

Let's look at the sequence Tricky Gary wants us to believe:

- Ancel Keys said we should eat X.
- Eisenhower ate X.
- Eisenhower died from a heart attack, despite eating X.
- Thus, Ancel Keys was wrong about eating X to prevent heart attacks.
- Therefore, ever since, the American Heart Association and everyone else has been wrong to tell us to eat X or to worry about cholesterol.

Step 2 - that "Eisenhower ate X"- (and all the illogic based on it) is pure, unadulterated hogwash. Anything less like Keys' diet than Eisenhower's is hard to imagine, yet Taubes has no problem pretending they're the same.

You probably have your own idea of what a Mediterranean diet is, and perhaps it's like mine - lots of grains and beans, fruits and vegetables, nuts and seeds, some fish, a little meat, some dairy and a fair amount of olive oil. Besides the fruit Ike stopped eating for breakfast when he threw his nutrition toys out the cot in 1958, where are the healthy fresh fruits and vegetables in Eisenhower's diet? Did Ancel Keys urge people to eat big salads with an olive oil and balsamic vinegar dressing, or did he tell us to eat fried junk? Margaret and Ancel Keys wrote another book in 1967 called *The Benevolent Bean*. How many times a week was Eisenhower eating legumes (which would have helped stave off his diabetes)?

The truth is this - Keys advised us to eat X, and Eisenhower ate Z.

Knowing that, where's the Eisenhower paradox Taubes is trying to foist on the credulous? The only paradox about Eisenhower and his diet isn't that he died so soon while eating a "low-fat, low-cholesterol, heart-healthy" diet. It's that he showed the (double-edged) resilience of our species which allowed him to eke out an existence for so long while eating so many animals and so much junk, and while eating almost no whole vegetables and fruits. The paradox is that he lived as long as he did as a Meater and Junker.

There's a Monty Python sketch called "The Funniest Joke in the World," which goes like this: "This man is Ernest Scribbler, writer of jokes. In a few moments, he will have written the funniest joke in the world and, as a consequence, he will die laughing." And that's exactly what happens. Ernest Scribbler laughs so hard he keels over dead. Then the joke he's written gets taken to the War Department, where they break it up into smaller, non-lethal sections, for translation into German. Allied soldiers, none of whom understand German, and with plugs in their ears, then chant the joke in unison as they march towards the German lines, but even so, many of them are badly injured because the joke is so powerful. The Germans, though, get the joke (which is funny in itself) and rise up from out of their trenches, laughing uproariously, then fall down dead.

That's how I feel about Gary Taubes's writing. Any more than two pages at a time would surely be the death of me, not from hilarity but from anger at his dishonesty, and the knowledge that his duplicity is killing the customers he betrays every day. To be fair, it's not just Taubes; it's most of the LCBAs and paleofantasists, and, if you can believe it, some of them are even worse than Taubes. As a prime specimen, I can only read a page of Tim Noakes a day, sometimes less. Sometimes my bullshit dosimeter tells me to take a week off to decontaminate after a single astonishingly loathsome sentence.

That's enough of Taubes for now. There's plenty more about him (and his devoted fan, Noakes) in *The Low-Carb Bullshit Artists Are Lying Us to Death*. Now let's go meet some other Low-Carb and Paleo Bullshit Artist(e)s…

The Meater Hall of Shame ~ Swindlers' List

Here are some high-animal diet proponents I've chosen for inclusion in a "Meater Hall of Shame," along with some of their writings. Not everyone in this list is a low-carber or a paleo advocate, and not all of them are liars. Some are just antediluvian folk who think animals can be part of a healthy diet. They're listed in chronological order of publication:

Anthelme Brillat-Savarin (1755 - 1826) - *The Physiology of Taste* (1825)

William Banting (1796 - 1878) - "Letter on Corpulence, Addressed to the Public" (1863)

William Harvey - *On Corpulence in Relation to Disease* (1872)

Vilhjalmur Stefansson (1879 - 1962) - *My Life with the Eskimo* (1913); *The Friendly Arctic* (1921); *The Fat of the Land* (1956)

Weston A. Price (1870 - 1948) - *Nutrition and Physical Degeneration* (1939)

John Yudkin (1910 - 1995) - *Pure, White, and Deadly* (1972), called *Sweet and Dangerous* in the USA.

Robert Atkins (1930 - 2003) - *Dr. Atkins' Diet Revolution* (1972); *Dr. Atkins' New Diet Revolution* (1999)

S. Boyd Eaton, MD and Melvin Konner PhD. Paleolithic Nutrition — A Consideration of Its Nature and Current Implications. *N Engl J Med* 1985.

S. Boyd Eaton (1938 -   ) - *The Paleolithic Prescription* (1988)

Michael Eades and Mary Dan Eades - *Protein Power* (1996)

Peter D'Adamo - *Eat Right 4 Your Type* (1996)

Andrew Weil (1942 -   ) - *8 Weeks to Optimum Health* (1997)

Patrick Holford - *The Optimum Nutrition Bible* (1997); *The New Optimum Nutrition Bible* (2004)

Sally Fallon and Mary Enig (1931 - 2014) - *Nourishing Traditions* (1999)

Pierre Dukan - *The Dukan Diet* (2000); *The Dukan Diet Made Easy* (2011)

Uffe Ravnskov (1934 -   ) - *The Cholesterol Myths* (2000); *Ignore the Awkward: How the Cholesterol Myths Are Kept Alive* (2010)

Loren Cordain (1950 -   ) - *The Paleo Diet* (2002)

Gary Taubes (1956 -   ) - "What if it's all been a big fat lie?" *NY Times* (7 July 2002); *Good Calories, Bad Calories* (2007), called *The Diet Delusion* outside the USA; *Why We Get Fat, and What to Do About It* (2010); The science of obesity: What do we really know about what makes us fat? *Br Med J* 2013.

Arthur Agatston (1947 -   ) - *The South Beach Diet* (2003)

Joseph Mercola (1954 -   ) - *The No-Grain Diet* (2003)

Jeff Volek - *Men's Health TNT Diet* (2007)

Malcolm Kendrick - *The Great Cholesterol Con* (2008)

Barry Sears - *The Zone* (2009)

Mark Sisson (1953 -   ) - *The Primal Blueprint* (2009); *Primal Endurance* (2016)

Robb Wolf - *The Paleo Solution* (2010)

Eric Westman, Stephen Phinney and Jeff Volek - *The New Atkins for a New You* (2010)

Arthur De Vany (1937 -   ) - *The New Evolution Diet* (2011)

Jeff Volek and Stephen Phinney - *The Art and Science of Low Carbohydrate Living* (2011); *The Art and Science of Low Carbohydrate Performance* (2012)

Robert Lustig - *Fat Chance* (2012)

Joel Salatin - *Folks, This Ain't Normal* (2012)

Jonny Bowden - *The Great Cholesterol Myth* (2012)

Eric Westman - *A Low Carbohydrate, Ketogenic Diet Manual* (2013)

David Perlmutter - *Grain Brain* (2013); *Brain Maker* (2015)

Denise Minger - *Death by Food Pyramid* (2013)

Jimmy Moore & Eric Westman - *Cholesterol Clarity* (2013); *Keto Clarity* (2014)

Anthony Colpo - *The Great Cholesterol Con* (2013)

Tim Noakes (1949 -   ) et al - *The Real Meal Revolution* (2013)

William Davis - *Wheat Belly* (2014)

Richard D. Feinman (1940 -   ) - *The World Turned Upside Down* (2014)

Nina Teicholz - *The Big Fat Surprise* (2014)

Bryan Walsh - Eat Butter. *Time* (23 June 2014)

Andreas Eenfeldt - *Low Carb, High Fat Food Revolution* (2014)

Mark Hyman (1959 -   ) - *The Blood Sugar Solution* (2014); *Eat Fat, Get Thin* (2016).

These are the people whose writings I dissect in *The Low-Carb Bullshit Artists Are Lying Us to Death*. We're done with the Who; let's look now at the How.

The Devil's Toolbox - How LCBAs get away with murdering us

Here are some of the 'lying tools' the Low-Carb and Paleo Bullshit Artists and other Meater apologists have at their disposal to try to bullshit us that animals are food, and which I describe more fully in the book wot I'm writing.

Lie#1: The False Dichotomy
Because junk causes an insulin spike in our blood, we should eat animals.

Lie #2: Reductionism
Avoiding The Big Picture of eating and health for all it's worth, because that shows an extremely high-whole-carb, no-animal diet to be the healthiest.

Lie #3: Euphemisms
Low-carb = high-animal, plus other veiled meanings. A peculiarity of "low-carbers" is that they don't define "carbs." Doing so gives the game away.

Lie #4: The veiled attack on Planting
The real foe for LCBAs isn't "low-fat" diets, it's Planting - eating nothing but whole plants.

Lie #5: Biological absurdity
The LCBAs' bizarre demonization of glucose and insulin. Plus their weird fringe belief that fat is our cells' primary fuel, not glucose. (Tim Noakes's assertion that "Of the three macronutrients in our diet, only carbohydrate is completely non-essential for life" is fatuous beyond belief. For one thing, for them to thrive, our gut flora *must* eat plenty of carbohydrate (and other plants-only nutrients). And as go our gut bacteria, so go we. They are us, we are them. What a nincompoop. I like that word - it fits Noakes to a T.)

Lie #5a: The internal contradiction
Animal protein evokes an insulin response, just like "carbs" do.

Lie #5b: The glycemic index
Index inventor Dr. David Jenkins isn't a low-carber; he's a high-carber.

Lie #6: The paleo lie
Animals aren't food, so paleo is The Big So What? Irrelevant to nutrition.

Lie #6a: "Design"
Paleofantasists call themselves scientists but love to use the D-word.

Lie#6b: The "grains are evolutionarily novel" lie vs. the animals are evolutionarily novel truth
Fewer than 1% of Planters who eat wheat suffer from celiac disease. 100% of people who eat animals develop a degree of atherosclerosis.

Lie #7: Americans became fat by eating a "low-fat" diet.
Other than Planters, no Americans have ever eaten a real low-fat diet.

Lie #8: Historical revisionism
Lying about the past. Look on with awe as Taubes and his bootleggers lie Eisenhower, Keys and Senator George McGovern out of all recognition.

Lie #9: Lies of commission
A.k.a. Making Stuff Up. Telling active lies, rather than Leaving Stuff Out.

Lie #10: Lies of omission
We saw Gary Taubes in action earlier, deftly combining multiple lies of omission with historical revision of Eisenhower's ill-health. He'd just embarked on the same dual makeover of Ancel Keys when we left him.

Lie #11a: Cherry picking
Picking and choosing what to put in, what to leave out… unethical behavior of which many LCBAs accuse nutrition legend Ancel Keys.

Lie #11b: Double standards about cherry picking
I devote a chapter of *Bullshit Artists* to resuscitating poor Keys, showing how LCBAs cherry pick data to falsely accuse Keys of cherry picking.

Lie #12: Lying by implication
Lying in such a way that you don't actually tell a porky pie but you leave a very strong impression that something is or isn't so.

Lie #13: Broad, sweeping (false) generalizations
Self-explanatory. Loren Cordain, e.g.: "It [the paleo diet] is the diet to which all of us are ideally suited." Er, dying young doesn't suit me, thanks, Loren.

Lie #14a: Drawing false conclusions from true premises
You're reading a paper, nodding your head in agreement, until – whoa! whiplash moment! – summary time arrives and the author concludes with something so at odds with what's gone before that your head whizzes around on your shoulders a few times like Linda Blair's in *The Exorcist*.

Lie #14b: Setting up a faulty premise so as to draw a false conclusion
Example: Siri-Tarino et al (2010) picked a bunch of bad studies to include in a meta-analysis of saturated fats, didn't find anything wrong there, so they reported that ALL saturated fats are fine. In effect: "(Because we weren't really trying to find it), we didn't find it, so it doesn't exist." Despicable.

Lie #15: Ad hominem or ad feminam arguments
Attacking people rather than their arguments. Big in the paleo blogosphere.

Lie #16: Using the whole truth to tell a lie OR "Cholesterol is vital for good health" [No shit, Sherlock]
Telling the truth about something in such a way that the implication is left that the people you're trying to discredit are total idiots for not knowing this most obvious of truths, whereas it's a given.

Lie #17: Using part of the truth to tell a lie
An example: feeding animal fat to people with very high cholesterol levels *cannot* raise their levels much - they're full. Concluding that animal fat *never* raises cholesterol is a lie - feed it to healthy people and their levels shoot up.

Lie #18: Unpublished data
Peter D'Adamo has spun this one out for decades, promising that he's just weeks or months away from unleashing the amazing results of his blood group diet studies upon an awe-struck world. Never gonna happen.

Lie #19: Unverifiable evidence: so-and-so said…
Expecting us to believe words a researcher said rather than what they wrote.

Lie #20: Taking stuff out of context
Taking what was said about one topic and misapplying it to another.

Lie #21: Misquoting
When Noakes and Mercola tell us that Otto Warburg said something about sugar and cancer, be sure to check 'cos Warburg says the exact opposite.

Lie #21a: Mangle a quote in print and leave us to read the complaints from your sources elsewhere
A Gary Taubes specialty. Not a few people he interviewed for his opening, cunningly titled salvo of low-carb lies - "What if it's all been a big fat lie?" (*NY Times* 2002) - were incensed by the way he misrepresented their views.

Lie #22: Substituting one word for another in a deceptive way

Peter "Praise the Lard" Attia can be pretty confusing when he talks about cholesterol, lipids and fats as if these words are interchangeable. Perhaps he thinks they are?

Lie #23: Distractionism

The magician flourishes one hand to divert us from what the other is doing.

Lie #23a: Cholesterol distractionism

Behaving as if cholesterol is the only potential problem with animals-as-food. It's not - it's one of dozens.

Lie #23b: Ancel Keys distractionism

A hybrid of cholesterol distractionism and historical revisionism… Behaving as if by (dishonestly) "debunking" a paper by Ancel Keys (dating back to 1953!) that the century-old cholesterol theory has been overturned. Effectively, they want us to believe that there've been no breakthroughs in lipidology in over 60 years, despite 13 Nobel Prizes being awarded to cholesterol researchers. Keys was a wonderful scientist, but not *indispensible* for Diet-Heart, or the lipid hypothesis, or the cholesterol theory, call it what you will, to achieve near-unanimous acceptance among educated scientists.

Lie #23b1: Brown-and-Goldstein obscurantism

A corollary of Ancel Keys distractionism. Low-Carb Bullshit Artists never, ever, ever, ever… ever discuss the work of Michael Brown and Joseph Goldstein, perhaps the greatest of all the cholesterol researchers.

They'd rather lie about Keys' 1953 "Atherosclerosis: a problem in newer public health" than try to take on B&G's 1985 Nobel acceptance speech, "A receptor-mediated pathway for cholesterol homeostasis." I, on the other hand, talk freely about B&G in *The Low-Carb Bullshit Artists Are Lying*…

Lie #23c: Sugar distractionism

Behaving as if because junk is bad for us (and it is), we should eat animals. LCBAs use junk as their universal scapegoat to exonerate Meating.

Lie #23d: Vitamin B$_{12}$ distractionism

The "It's-not-in-a-plants-only-diet-so-a-plants-only-diet-must-be-bad" hokum; meaning, we should eat animals because of their B$_{12}$ contamination.

Lie #23e: Essential Meater nutrients distractionism

The "It's-in-animals-so-it-must-be-a-nutrient" bulldust, as applied to such metabolites as choline, carnitine, creatine and long-chain fatty acids.

Lie #23f: Weight loss distractionism

Behaving as if weight loss is the be-all and end-all of nutrition. Meating to lose weight when Planting does it better and more healthily makes no sense.

Lie #23f1: Eating animals provides a "metabolic advantage"

Eating animals is simply inefficient. It requires more energy to turn fat into glucose for fuel (gluconeogenesis) than simply to eat glucose-packed plants.

Lie #23f2: Eating lots of animals causes satiety

Planters feel sated or satiated after a meal because our stomachs' stretch receptors tell our brains we've eaten enough bulky fiber, and our gastric nutrient receptors say that we've received enough nutrients. Because animals and other junk are fiber- and nutrient-deficient, these two mechanisms don't work for Meaters. They think they're sated out of repulsion: their bodies cry Hold! Enough already of this fat and protein rubbish. Planting is about feeding our cells; Meating is about starving them. Planting is anabolic; Meating is catabolic… and catastrophic.

Lie #24: Repeating old, outdated stuff *ad nauseam*

A much-used Meater ploy, especially about omega-3 fats from fishes. The obsession with long-chain fats dates back to the '80s when the DART study found them beneficial. DART-2, a later, bigger, better study, overturned that verdict. Fish oil is big business. DART-1 is where the money is.

Lie #25: Ancient studies

LCBAs love ooooooooooooollllllllllddddddddddddd studies - Ancel Keys, c. 1953? You got it. Otto Warburg, 1930s? Done. And then they still lie about them! I know - I've read the original papers, and I'll show you them.

Lie #26: Anachronisms

Getting the time sequence wrong. For example, scienceofnutrition.com's Seth Yoder reports that on page 23 of *The Big Fat Surprise*, Nina Teicholz says that a 1992 paper was refuted by a later paper which came out in 1985. The Keys bashers out there who tell us that two guys called Yerushalmy and Hilleboe smashed what Tim Noakes refers to as Keys' "false doctrine" in 1957 must marvel at Y&H's prescience, seeing as Keys published his first paper on his epic Seven Countries Study 13 years later, in 1970.

Lie #27: Dead people

Omnia nisi bonum. LCBAs love to speak ill of the dead, free from reprisal. Ancel Keys, Otto Warburg, George McGovern et al.

Lie #28: Young people
References to positions taken by scientists early in their careers, leaving the impression that their later, more mature incarnations agree with them.

Lie #29: Straw people
Called "straw man studies" in the old, pre-PC days, they're a favorite of LCBAs. They're studies which claim to be something they're not, and when you knock them down, you claim you knocked down the other thing. I'll show you half a dozen comparisons of low-carb diets against - nudge nudge, wink wink - "low-fat" diets which turn out to be high-fat diets. (Noakes has 5 of them in his squalid book.)

Lie #30: Wrong people
Duping the public by citing studies long discarded as bullshit by anyone with the least education in nutrition.

Lie #31: Sick people
Talking the talk, not walking the walk. A discussion of some of the heart-diseased and diabetic LCBAs who presume to give health advice to others. Price, Atkins and Noakes spring to mind.

Lie #32: Fat people
Do as I say, not as I do. A discussion of the many overweight and obese LCBAs who presume to give weight loss advice to others. A long list.

Lie #33: Fictional people
Using characters from literature as if they represent the views of their authors. A Taubes forté.

Lie#34: Lying people
Copying known liars is never a good idea - Teicholz, Noakes and others pilfering from Taubes without checking up on Taubes… bad career move.

Lie #35: Industry-funded people
Hired gun researchers almost never bite the hand that feeds them. (That would be like killing the goose that lays the golden eggs.)

Lie 35a: Independent researchers
Westman, Phinney and Volek may think of themselves as independent researchers. I'm curious why the book they co-wrote, *The New Atkins for a New You*, is "copyright © 2010 by Atkins Nutritionals, Inc." Were W, P & V employees or independent authors on this Atkins puff piece project?

Lie #36: Good all-rounders
Leonardos of lying, polymaths of perjury, liars so accomplished that they bestride the thoroughfares of lying like colossi of crooked roads. Good all-rounders are conversant with all the tools in the Devil's Toolbox.

Lie #37: Ignoring the evidence of our eyes
Mere observation shows Planters to be the healthiest and longest-lived people in the world, as in the famous Blue Zones where *high-carb* diets rule, but who you gonna believe - the LCBAs or your lying eyes?

Lie #38a: "Correlation isn't causation"
Who knew? If someone tells us "correlation isn't causation," run. They're trying to kill us by bullshitting us that all the correlations (along with their explanatory "plausible biological mechanisms") showing the harms of Meating are meaningless.

Lie #38b: Double standards: epidemiology (population studies)
LCBAs hate epidemiology, because it makes them look stupid, yet they use really bad population studies when it suits them. A Noakes forté.

Lie #39: Double standards: case control studies
LCBAs like Nina Teicholz say they can't abide case control studies, because of "recall bias": people can't reliably remember what they ate. Fair enough, but then you shouldn't turn around and use them when they suit your purpose, dear Nina, as you do in *The Big Fat Surprise*.

Lie #40: Unusual people – outing the liars about the outliers
Somehow, to LCBAs, despite a heap of confounding factors, studies of Maasai or Inuit health are more relevant to our health than studies of our health.

Lie #41: "Mistaking the map for the territory"
Substituting photos of the Mona Lisa for the real deal.

Lie #41a: Biomarkers vs. outcomes
Telling us that lowering our A1c or Tc levels - or whatever - is more important than reversing heart disease. Only Planting does both.

Lie #41b: Soft end points
Hard end points are real health outcomes; soft are possible stations along the way. Which would you prefer? Which do you think the LCBAs favor? Here's your answer: JS Volek, MJ Sharman, CE Forsythe: Modification of lipoproteins by very low-carbohydrate diets. *J Nutr* 2005, 135(6):1339-1342.

Meaters "modify lipoproteins" while Planters like Ornish reverse heart disease. Low-Carb Bullshit Artists are Neros fiddling while Rome burns.

Lie #42: Lack of references
Our default mode should be to assume that any unreferenced statement by an LCBA is probably a lie or, to be charitable, untrue.

Lie #42a: Check those references
Hell, many of the LCBAs' *referenced* statements are untrue. They don't say what they say they do. As Ronald Reagan almost said: "[Don't] trust, but [definitely] verify." Examples abound.

Lie #43: Ignoring good science
Ignoring entire landmark studies, not just parts of them, as in lies of omission. For instance, there's an amazing Finnish study showing how Finns gained 6 to 7 extra years of life [!!] by converting dairies into berry farms. That's a stupendous result, about which the LCBAs keep schtum.

Lie #44: Substituting bogus low carb bullshit for great studies
I give examples of brilliant, life-saving science which the Low-Carbers don't respond to but instead counter with the most putrescent garbage, such as a deceptive blogpost telling us "The Swedes Are Eating More Butter!" [Poor Swedes.] The difference in the evidentiary value of this high-animal bullshit to #43 above shows how desperate the LCBAs are becoming.

Lie #45a: Scientific method – The low-carbers' ayes
LCBAs deliberately choose the types of scientific studies that are the worst sorts of studies for gathering nutrition information. They love useless cross-sectional studies. They love studies of homogeneous populations. They like autopsy studies. They love single nutrient studies. They love to measure (deceptive) fasting cholesterol levels, many hours after the inflammatory, oxidative damage has been done, which is kind of like a traffic cop pulling over a drunk and getting him to take a breathalyzer test the following morning, after a good night's sleep. They adore randomized, placebo-controlled, double-blind, cross-over studies, as if the individual nutrients in foods are drugs, rather than parts of a synergistic whole known as food.

Lie #45a1: Reliance on self-reported studies
Telling us, as Tim Noakes does, that subjects *self-reported* weight loss "among the largest yet described" is to be "not even wrong." Contemptible.

Lie #45b: Scientific method – the low-carbers' nays

The corollary of Lie #45a – avoiding the best evidence.

As we've seen, LCBAs hate epidemiology/population studies, especially when there's a wide variation in diets and outcomes, which is extremely useful. They never study whole foods. They shun migration studies. They can't stand twin studies. They never test low-carb diets against a proper vegan diet, only a pale shadow of it. In fact, they loathe all the studies that are the best ways to find useful, thought-provoking… *correlations* (I know. Don't say it…) between dietary inputs and health outcomes.

Why do they ac-cent the negative, and e-lim-inate the positive in their perversion of the scientific method, the low-carbers? By now you know the answer. They're not interested in the truth - they're bullshit artists.

Lie #46: Ignore-ance or Ignorance of exciting new scientific fields

To be thought credible by the credulous, the LCBAs+Ps must "deny" entire fields of science. Think: epidemiology, cardiology, lipidology. Here are some new ones:

Lie #46a: I&I of Microbiomics

Microbiomics is the study of our gut flora which shows how Meating is still 'evolutionarily novel' and harmful; and how Planting benefits us.

Lie #46b: I&I of Epigenetics

The science of epigenetics shows how Meating brings out the worst in our genetic code, and Planting the best.

Lie #46c: I&I of Nutrigenomics

Nutrigenomics - what we could call Applied Epigenetics - shows how we can use nutrition epigenetically, to beneficially express our genes through Planting or to cause havoc through Meating.

Dean Ornish showed how Planting up- and down-regulates hundreds of genes to help cure prostate cancer. (Not improve biomarkers; *cure*.)

Lie #47: Starting your own NPO to promote trash science

The Nutrition & Metabolism Society is an advocacy group for low-carbism, a not-for-profit organization with tax-exempt status to help kill us.

Lie #48: Starting your own journal to publish trash science

A.k.a. Dodging peer review by substituting dodgy peer review.

Nutrition & Metabolism is the N&M Society's online journal for low-carbism. Here are some people who've served on its editorial board: Michael Eades, Richard Feinman, Eugene Fine, Stephen Phinney, Jeff Volek, Eric

Westman, Richard Wood and William Yancy. Nothing but Low-Carb and Paleo Bullshit Artists as far as the eye can see. "Water, water everywhere; Nor any drop to drink."

Lie #49: Starting your own research center to perform trash science
With a reported $40 million in hand, the Nutrition Science Initiative (NuSI) say they're going to perform studies comparing the low-carb [high-animal] diet to… brace yourself… the Standard American Diet.

Wow.

Ow.

GIGO = Garbage In, Garbage Out.

These are the Limbo Dancers of Nutrition - no matter how low Gary Taubes and Peter Attia set the bar for themselves, they manage to slither under it.

Lie #50: Making up organizations to reference
PlantPositive is pretty funny about this. He shows Peter Attia, Gary Taubes's partner in grime at NuSI, providing a reference, complete with graphic, from something he calls the USFAO. Just like FAO Schwarz's legendary 5th Avenue toy store, the USFAO doesn't exist. Unlike FAO Schwarz 5th Avenue, it never did.

Bonus lie# 51: Nutritionists are full of it
If there's one qualification that LCBAs and paleonutters seem absolutely to despise in their quest for mastery of nutrition science, it's even the most rudimentary education or certification in… nutrition science. Sports physiologists, English majors who once took a course in statistics, ex-journalists, physicians, undertakers, gourmands and anthropologists abound, but trained nutritionists are like hen's teeth in low-carbland. Go figure.

The truth is that, just as in any other science, almost 100% of the best work in nutrition and other biomedical sciences comes from within these disciplines, not from untutored outsiders, as the mostly untutored Low-Carb outsiders would have us believe.

Genius outsiders like Einstein (who worked for a while as a Patent Examiner in the Swiss patent office) do sometimes move into academia and revolutionize entire sciences, as Einstein did with physics, but for every hundred wannabe Einsteins in the world of low-carb (or a Copernicus, even, as one double-barreled dolt hilariously called Tim Noakes), there appears to be only one lab assistant who knows where the light switch is.

And let me remind Meaters that Einstein - often considered a classic Thomas Kuhn outsider - championed a vegan diet near the end of his life.

Putting in 10,000 hours of practice at eating animals doesn't make us Gladwellian experts in the ideal way to eat.

So, that's it… The Devil's Toolbox of Low-Carb Lying Techniques, my conditional rendering thereof, *The Low-Carb Bullshit Artists Are Lying Us to Death* being a work in progress due for publication later in 2016.

Please feel free to send me your favorite "terminological inexactitudes" by your favorite Low-Carb Bullshit Artist, especially if you've identified a double-dealing category I've missed. Ta.

Late-breaking lie #52: Highfalutin chapter heading quotes

Another Taubes forté. A sly way to create a false impression of truthfulness is to begin your chapters with a pretentious quote, the more obscure the better. For example, Taubes starts Chapter 3 of *Good Calories, Bad Calories*, "The Creation of Consensus," with a quote from Francis Bacon's *Novum Organum* (1620): "In sciences that are based on supposition and opinion… the object is to command assent, not to master the thing itself." Is nutrition a science based on "supposition and opinion?" No, it's no less evidence-based than any other, but Taubes wants us to think it is.

(By the way, Bacon also said: "Some books are to be tasted, others to be swallowed, and some few to be chewed and digested." And some, like Taubes's, should play no part in our diets.)

To open Part Two: The Carbohydrate Hypothesis, Taubes uses a farcical quote by CC and SM Furnas from their authoritative-sounding *Man, Bread & Destiny: The Story of Man and His Food* (1937): "If the proportion of carbohydrates is high then the amount of something else of greater importance is low." Bwa ha ha. Pure claptrap. Putting its name in lights up on the marquee doesn't make it any less crapulous. You can stick lipstick on a porky pie… but it's still a lie.

Okay, pig, that'll do with the lying techniques, that'll do.

Finally, here's the book outline, as it looks today, to round out this preview of *The Low-Carb Bullshit Artists Are Lying Us to Death*:

Outline - *The Low-Carb Bullshit Artists Are Lying Us to Death*

Chapter 1: Why the Low-Carb Bullshit Artists tell porky pies
Because of the rapidly emerging biomedical consensus in favor of Planting, and against Meating and Junking, Low-Carb Bullshit Artists have no choice but to tell lies. Meaters lack any credible science to back their outdated idea of animals-as-food. Readers of *Why Animals Aren't Food* will understand why.

To confirm that animals aren't food for human beings, I give a brief description of what's in various animal items and the damage that eating them causes: "red" flesh, poultry, eggs, dairy and fishes.

Chapter 2: The Meater Hall of Shame
A history of the low-carb and paleo shtick from the 18th Century to the present. The lineage or intellectual heritage, as it were, of low-carb, as selected by low-carbers themselves (but not as they've described them): from fat Anthelme Brillat-Savarin to fat William Banting to fat, heart-diseased Weston A. Price and so on… until the rise of the modern psychopaths - obese, heart-diseased Robert Atkins and his foul brood.

Chapter 3: Modern Times - The Artful Dodger
Parajournalist Gary Taubes shows us how it's done. Commentary on his dodgy treatment of Leo Tolstoy, Benjamin Spock, Dwight David Eisenhower, Ancel Keys, George McGovern and Dean Ornish.

Chapter 4: Scraping Taubes's Shit Off Our Shoes, Part 1
A short biography of Ancel Keys, restoring the reputation of a Giant of Nutrition.

Chapter 5: Scraping Taubes's Shit From Between Our Toes, Part 2
The real story of Senator George McGovern and the US Dietary Guidelines.

Chapter 6: Plagiarism is the sincerest form of flattery
Some of the Low-Carb Bullshit Artists who've swallowed and regurgitated-without-digesting Taubes's codswallop about Keys and others, especially two of Keys' 'opponents,' Jacob Yerushalmy and Herman Hilleboe. The P-for-plagiarism word pops up. Plenty.

Chapter 7: The Devil's Toolbox
A description of more than 50 lying techniques the LCBAs use to get away with murdering us, with copious examples of who said what to whom.

Chapter 8: And the Winner Is…

In which I have a hard time deciding which of the Low-Carb Bullshit Artists has said or written the stupidest thing about a nutrition-related topic - there's stiff competition between Uffe Ravnskov, Chris Masterjohn, Tim Noakes, Sally-Ann Creed, Denise Minger, Joel Salatin and Robert Lustig. (Oh, hell's bells, all of them.)

Chapter 8: The Worst Book Ever Written?

An in-depth discussion of *The Real Meal Revolution* (2013), a fetid turd of a book by Tim Noakes, Sally-Ann Creed, Jonno Proudfoot and David Grier. There's a spectacular stupidity or a shameful lie on every page Noakes writes in this verkakte book, including the front cover. Even the title is a lie to those of us who know *Why Animals Aren't Food.*

Chapter 9: Look Back in Amazement, Look Forward with Tranquility

An explanation of why and how these Lying Sacks of Shit have gotten away with their lying lies for so long. And why, as compassionate eater Mahatma Gandhi said: "When I despair, I remember that all through history the way of truth and love have always won. There have been tyrants and murderers [just like the Low-Carb Bullshit Artists and the Paleofantasists], and for a time, they can seem invincible, but in the end, they always fall. Think of it - always."

"The way of truth and love" in nutrition is… Planting - eating nothing but whole fruits and vegetables (and taking our vitamin B_{12}). Planting, like music, "has Charms to sooth a savage Breast, To soften Rocks, or bend a knotted Oak." Planting has the power to mend almost anything, even the fools' catastrophe inflicted by Meating and Junking.

I live in a literary 'hard hat zone.' *The Low-Carb Bullshit Artists Are Lying Us to Death* is a work under construction, and it probably won't retain its present form. My hope is that this intro and projected outline and The Devil's Toolbox of low-carb and paleo lying techniques will help you to identify and evade the wide array of tools the Low-Carb Bullshit Artists use to lie us to death about animals-as-food.

Remember: animals are not food. That's all we need to know to keep ourselves and our loved ones safe from the ravages of sad, mad or bad Meaterialists when they try to foist dead animals upon us.

I wrote *Why Animals Aren't Food* because I had to - I couldn't find a comprehensive anthology of the nutrition science showing the ill-effects of eating animals. We needed one badly.

And I'm writing *The Low-Carb Bullshit Artists Are Lying Us to Death* for the same reason. We need to know all we can about these unscrupulous and ignorant thieves of our health.

"Things reveal themselves passing away," wrote W.B. Yeats: we get to see hidden realities when they're almost gone. Meating is on its way out, and low-carb and paleo diets are two of the Meaters' desperate, last-ditch, rearguard actions to try to prevent their warped ideology from being obliterated by the growing consensus of Planting's supremacy. Bad science, PR and lies are the only tools the Low-Carb Bullshit Artists have.

The intrinsic dishonesty of the low-carb (and other reactionary, counter-revolutionary, animal-eating) anti-scientists is an important topic about which no one has yet written a book that covers it in the depth it deserves. There are probably a few million people on Planet A who're better qualified than I am to write these books, but as Melvin (the character played by Jack Nicholson in *As Good As It Gets*) says to the startled people waiting in his shrink's anteroom: "What if this is as good as it gets?"

For all our sakes, I pray that PlantPositive breaks cover one day soon and comes out to moider da bums in print. Till then, all apologies, dear hearts - I'm it and, for now, this is as good as it gets.

So long, and thanks for not eating all the fishes.

Rohan Millson
Greyton Farm Animal Sanctuary
Western Cape
South Africa
5 April 2016

Printed in Great Britain
by Amazon

16000499R00138